LOSE IT RIGHT

A Brutally Honest,
3-Stage Program to
Help You Get Fit
and Lose Weight
Without Losing Your Mind

James S. Fell

and Margaret Yúfera-Leitch, PhD

In consultation with Lindy Kennedy, MSc., RD

RANDOM HOUSE CANADA

PUBLISHED BY RANDOM HOUSE CANADA

Copyright © 2014 James Fell

www.randomhouse.ca

Random House Canada and colophon are registered trademarks.

This book is intended as a reference volume only and not as a medical manual. It is not intended
as a substitute for any treatment that may have been prescribed by a doctor. The author is not
responsible for your specific health or allergy needs that may require medical supervision, or for
any adverse reactions to the recipes contained in this book.

The recommendations in this book are generic, since nutritional needs vary depending on age,
sex, and health status. If you suspect that you have a serious medical problem, the author strongly
recommends seeking proper medical treatment.

Library and Archives Canada Cataloguing in Publication

Fell, James, 1968–
　　　Lose it right : a brutally honest 3-stage program to help you get fit and lose weight without
losing your mind / James Fell and Margaret Yúfera-Leitch.

Includes index.
Also issued in electronic format.

ISBN 978-0-345-81246-9

　　　1. Physical fitness. 2. Weight loss. 3. Exercise. 1. Nutrition. I. Yúfera-Leitch, Margaret
II. Title.

RA781.F445 2014　　　　613.7　　　　C2013-900749-0

Cover and text design by Leah Springate

Cover image: Lori Andrews

Printed and bound in the United States of America

10　9　8　7　6　5　4　3　2　1

Advance praise for **Lose It Right**

"After I quit bike racing I imperceptibly put on 15 pounds in a decade. But then I expected to lose them all in a couple of months. When that didn't happen I got discouraged and gave up. Now I understand why and what I need to do thanks to James Fell's firm but fair program to lose it right, keep it off, and shed my guilt along with my pounds. In an ocean of diet books, *Lose It Right* is the most rational and reasonable one I've read."

> Michael Shermer, publisher of *Skeptic* magazine, monthly columnist for *Scientific American*, author of *The Believing Brain*

"Reading a weight loss book can virtually never be described as entertaining, but then again, most weight loss books don't have James Fell as an author! With his trademark brash and often laugh-out-loud funny writing style, James and his co-author Margaret combine humor and evidence to provide a useable and science-based blueprint to inspire beginners and experts alike to be healthier, happier and more fit."

> Yoni Freedhoff, MD, author of *The Diet Fix*

"James Fell has just done everyone a favor. In heroic fashion without regard for his own safety, Fell jumps into the $70 billion a year tub of crap known as 'the weight loss industry.' Sifting through all the foul-smelling nonsense he separates the gimmicks most experts try to sell you and identifies the most realistic and sensible approach to long-term weight loss. If your goal is to achieve a healthy weight for the rest of your life with intelligent advice, read this book."

> Paul Plakas, Fitness Expert on Gemini Award–winning shows *Taking It Off* and *X-Weighted*

"You will learn and laugh out loud. An outstanding book that will engage you right away with its straight talk, clarity and practical applications derived from latest research. Essential reading for anybody interested in losing weight today."

> Miguel Alonso-Alonso, MD, Instructor in Neurology, Harvard Medical School

"James Fell has written a truly engaging, pragmatic and epiphanic book. *Lose It Right* is not just a healthy lifestyle plan that you do, but a person you become."

Sue D. Pedersen, MD, FRCP(C), Specialist in Endocrinology and Metabolism, C-ENDO Clinic, Calgary

"James Fell says his book *Lose It Right* is not a weight-loss book or 'get in shape' book but a lifestyle overhaul book. What he doesn't say is his book is easy to read and entertaining; funny yet factual; informative but inspirational. *Lose It Right* is the perfect book for the person who has failed at fad diets and now wants to learn how to manage food, weight and exercise for the long run. Fell will take you on a journey that is based on science, but couched in reality—along with a good dose of humor."

Nancy Clark, MS, RD, author of
Nancy Clark's Sports Nutrition Guidebook

International law dictates that I dedicate my first book to my wife.
In compliance, this one's for the lovely Dr. Heidi Fell.

CONTENTS

A NOTE FROM JAMES S. FELL

Margaret Yúfera-Leitch and I bonded over Oprah.

I wrote an "Open Letter to Oprah" for my fitness column in the *Los Angeles Times*. In it, I told Ms. Winfrey I thought her health and nutrition gurus were not helping. Margaret sent me an email, all the way from Spain, to tell me she thought the column was awesome.

Then I met Margaret, and I thought she was awesome. She's a respected obesity researcher with a *real* PhD in psychology from a *real* university. The focus of her studies has been eating behaviors and their link to body weight.

We bonded over Oprah . . . and our mutual disdain for the mass of male bovine droppings scattered all over the weight loss industry. This book represents our desire to bring sanity and honesty to an industry sorely lacking in both.

"You're not a real journalist until someone threatens to sue you."

An editor once said this to me. It was comforting at the time, because the person doing the threatening was a famous "weight loss guru." Our war of words made international news. And by "international" I mean they even covered it in the Ethiopian press.

That column led to much fan mail, moderate hate mail, and one threat to "cave [my] head in with a kettlebell."

Although I've made enemies through my writing about fitness and health, I've also made friends. World-renowned obesity researchers have sung my praises and shared my work, and I've lost count of how many medical doctors have told me they recommend my writing to their patients.

In *Lose It Right*, Margaret and I have distilled the best of our combined knowledge of healthy weight loss into a guide you can use in your own life. We've come up with a three-stage program that will help transform your eating behaviors and your lifestyle to create a leaner, healthier and higher-performing you. No miracles, secrets or magic; we rely on science and big-picture planning to help you achieve your goals.

Final warning: take note of the words "brutally" and "honest" in the subtitle.

Okay. Now that all the wimps are gone, let's do this.

INTRODUCTION

The first principle is that you must not fool yourself—
and you are the easiest person to fool.
　　—RICHARD FEYNMAN, Nobel laureate in physics

Here is part of a rejection letter I received in the early days of pitching this book, sent to my agent from the editor of a major publishing house:

> *There's so much I really like here, David. James has a brash*
> *and audacious voice, and a sensible and straightforward mes-*
> *sage. His column in the LA Times is great, and I like the way*
> *he approaches the material . . . But my main concern, I hate*
> *to admit, is the sensible, measured nature of his program.*
> *Despite his flashy prose, he actually writes like the informed*
> *journalist that he is . . . sane, levelheaded, with proven advice.*
> *And while that's great journalism, I worry that it's not salable*
> *as a diet plan.*

And people wonder why they can't lose weight.

EMPOWER THIS

I know how it goes: your boss is channeling Linda Blair to the point that you're waiting for the green vomit to fly, your kids are whining that they have so much homework it qualifies as a hate crime, the dog won't stop peeing on the rug, your in-laws are coming for a visit, the toilet seat got left up and you fell in.

   ·   Life keeps serving up lemons that someone fished out of a Dumpster until you want to start main-lining Häagen-Dazs and plowing through a bag of Doritos as if the apocalypse is imminent.

The food environment has programmed you to glue your butt to the couch and scarf pizza dipped in chocolate sauce because today sucked, but it doesn't have to be this way. There are real, science-based approaches to behavior change that are not the fluff and nonsense spouted by some Oprah-endorsed "emotional eating guru" whose qualifications amount to *been there, done that*.

Sorry, but no amount of group hugging or "empowerment" is going to help change your eating behaviors. There is no quick and easy way to learn to control what you consume. Following a calorie-conscious and nutritious diet is not comfortable at first, especially since we have 24/7 access to hyper-yummy junk food. And yes, resisting the sugar-coated grease blobs and making wise food choices is a skill that must be learned, because we're not evolutionarily programmed to instinctively know what's best for us to eat. Being toilet trained isn't a natural instinct either; I'd argue it's worth the effort.

Getting in shape is also worth the effort. *You* are worth the effort.

It's going to take effort.

Here's why: evolution programmed us to be fat storers. Most of the inherently skinny cavemen and women got naturally "selected out" as tasty treats for carrion eaters millennia ago. Those of us who stuck around, genetically speaking, got saddled with brains wired to crave pleasurable food. We also share the common trait of not wanting to be active if it isn't critical to survival. We're all about conserving those hard-earned and much-needed fat stores. Even today, our bodies are planning for the next big famine. (If evolution talk offends you, imagine that your ancestors rode dinosaurs and all of this happened only six thousand years ago.)

In a nutshell, this is what Stone Age people thought about diet and exercise:

SO HUNGRY—MUST STUFF FOOD IN FACE HOLE!

DON'T MOVE EXCEPT HUNT OR FLEE
SABER-TOOTHED MURDER BEAST!

Today, that mentality hasn't changed much; it's locked in our genes. But the problem is that now we have *much more* than all the food we need—and it tastes so good—and there is even less motivation to get off our expanding butt cheeks, because somebody invented the grocery store and machines do our labor for us. Most of us bitch if the drive-through window is closed, and the only place we see a murder beast is on the National Geographic Channel.

In other words, circumstances used to watch our waistlines for us, and circumstances have changed.

SKEPTICISM CAN MAKE YOU STRONG

Our troglodyte DNA wants us to be fat, so how do you combat your genes to get and stay slim? First, you must become skeptical of all things weight loss. It's a dirty, dirty industry full of male bovine droppings promising quick and easy results.

I am a shovel.

Who wants to lose weight slowly? That's lame. It's got to be *fast, dammit!* Guess what happens when I google "lose weight fast"? I get almost 10 million results and ads that include words such as "magic" and "miracle," plus Dr. Oz flogging octopus spleens to burn belly fat, or something. Then I google "lose weight slowly" and get only 13,000 results (and no ads), and most talk about things like "how to lose weight with a slow metabolism" or "to lose weight, slow your eating." Not the same thing.

Losing weight fast doesn't happen except in cases of significant obesity, but everyone—even if they are only a little overweight—*really wants it to be possible.* And the weight loss marketers take that desire and warp it, package it up all pretty and ram it down your throat via a massive deluge of advertising/brainwashing that permeates our society via every possible media outlet, often using celebrities, because . . .

SEX SELLS SLIMNESS

If you have an Internet connection and poor impulse control, you know why Kim Kardashian is famous. One hint: it's not for her knowledge of pharmacology. This is why I was surprised to see her on *20/20* talking about QuickTrim diet pills, which she and her sisters endorse. "We helped formulate this," she said.

Really? And that's a selling point?

And Kim wasn't just talking about diet pills. She also flogged Skechers Shape-Ups—the shoes that allegedly burn extra calories and tone your butt. That's the same Skechers, by the way, that agreed to pay $40 million to settle a class action lawsuit for false advertising.

If you want to know how to achieve "celebrity" as a result of a leaked sex tape, Kim is the one to look to. When it comes to the intricacies of sustainable weight loss for the population at large, however, I am suspicious of her qualifications.

WEIGHT LOSS INC.

Welcome to Weight Loss Inc., where serpent lubrication sells like hotcakes. It's capitalism run amok, and it is not helping. Weight Loss Inc. spends billions to perpetuate the myth of "quick and easy" when it comes to dropping fat from your frame. They do this because it's profitable. If you believe in quick-fix miracle cures for getting in shape, you're not alone. In 2011 the Federal Trade Commission launched a massive survey of consumer fraud in the United States and found that people were more likely to be taken in by a weight loss scam than any other type of fraud.[1] It's not all "bank inspectors" and pyramid schemes; year after year, fraudsters scam millions of Americans wanting to lose weight by selling pills, powders, machines, wraps, creams and even "weight loss earrings." Huh.

Are people who believe such things stupid? Not necessarily.

In his 1997 book *Why People Believe Weird Things,* Skeptics Society founder Michael Shermer asserted that "smart people" could be more susceptible to outrageous claims than others "because they are skilled at defending beliefs they arrived at for non-smart reasons." These non-smart reasons can include peer pressure, sibling and parental influences, life experiences, cultural pressure and even genetic predispositions. Shermer further explained: "More than any other, the reason people believe weird things is that they want to. It feels good. It is comforting. It is consoling."[2]

I had a chat with Shermer to get weight-loss-specific details.

"Weight loss is so susceptible for fraud because it's so hard to do and the signs of progress so slow," Shermer told me. "The reward is not enough for most people. Anything that appeals to shortening the process is going to sell."

Shermer, a competitive cyclist for 30 years, admits he's struggled himself. "The cost in difficulty for weight loss is very high, and for the average person it seems impossible." And so people spend money on weight loss "miracles" instead. "It's called the optimism bias," he said. "There are just enough success stories—either real or imagined—that people believe they will be the one who is successful." And they buy again and again because they have a poor memory for failure.

Sensationalism sells. Just look at Oprah, Dr. Phil or Dr. Oz and the guests they have on their shows. Extolling sustained weight loss that comes via a slow and steady approach with gradual integration of exercise and dietary restriction just isn't sexy, but "six-second abs" and magical raspberry ketones are. We have authors claiming it takes "eight minutes in the morning," that you can get a "Four-Hour Body," or that you should go on a "17-Day Diet," and these books and products become best sellers. There is no shortage of profiteers taking advantage of the obesity epidemic by pushing gimmicks and scams on a desperate populace. (This doesn't mean there isn't good stuff out there too; we will make recommendations.) We like to believe in the myth of the quick fix, because, as Shermer says, it's comforting.

Question: When has anything worthwhile in your life come about without serious and sustained effort?

If you want to lose fat and be healthy—if you want to get and *stay* in shape—it's going to take effort from now until the day you dirt nap. There is NO quick fix. There are no miracle cures. This will take both exercise (*ooh, scary!*) and dietary control, and you won't transform into a bikini model in a month. Deep down, you know that if something sounds too good to be true, it's about as reliable as choosing Lindsay Lohan as your designated driver.

I think that's about enough doom and gloom for now. Sustained weight loss *is* feasible. Here's how to lose it right.

LEARN, PREPARE, DO

You know how Nike says, "Just do it"? Well, they're wrong. You know what you get when you try to turn into a fitness fanatic overnight? A you-shaped bag of pain that thinks exercise sucks.

Don't "just do it." Instead, learn, prepare, *then do it*. This book helps you progress through all three stages. Stage I, Learn, will tell you everything you need to know about how your body works, how it reacts to food and how exercise is an invaluable tool for slimming down and getting fit. In Stage II, Prepare, we'll get you ready to embrace the lifestyle changes necessary for sustainable, long-term success. Finally, in Stage III, Do, you'll be introduced to the Virtuous Cycle, a leveled eating and exercise program that will gradually transform your health, the way your body performs and the way you look.

This program takes you through behavior change at a gradual pace you can tolerate. See those "MBA" letters after my name in my bio? I'm going to proactively synergize your core competencies toward an optimized fitness paradigm. Uh, I mean, this book is about designing a personal and comprehensive strategy for losing weight and getting fit, because some product you bought from an infomercial isn't going to change your physique or your life in just a few weeks.

You don't build a house by slapping a few boards together. You need a blueprint; you must lay a foundation and have the right skills, tools and building products. It takes teamwork. There are goals—both short and long term—to be set, tactics to be devised, time to be managed and schedules to be adhered to.

When you're building a house, quitting halfway through is not a great idea. However, this is okay when it comes to getting in shape. In other words, don't adopt the all-or-nothing mentality. If you think losing 50 pounds will make you fitness-model lean, but instead manage to maintain 25 pounds of weight loss, is this not still awesome? You get leaner, healthier, have more energy and drive. You've adopted an improved lifestyle you can live with and sustain. Yes, still awesome.

You can hold firm partway through the process if you're happy with your new lifestyle and the results you've achieved. We're not cracking whips but encouraging sustainable improvement.

But know that going from a metaphorical doughnut-scarfing couch potato to diet-conscious workout warrior—or even getting to the half-way point—is a serious undertaking. It's a big project, and in the business world you break big projects down into manageable pieces and complete them in a logical order.

The simple advice of "eat less, move more" is a crock. As we've seen, both evolution and the current environment are conspiring against us. Two-thirds of the population is overweight or obese because it's become too easy to gain weight, and too hard to get and stay slim. Saying "eat less, move more" to an overweight person is like saying "spend less, earn more" to someone living in crushing poverty. Granted, losing weight does require you to consume fewer calories and add physical activity, but learning how to integrate this into your life can't be boiled down to a sound bite.

We're going to make you somewhat uncomfortable one step at a time using our Virtuous Cycle exercise and eating plan. When each new step—each new behavior—becomes comfortable (or at least tolerable) and routine, it's time to get a little uncomfortable again. These baby steps reinforce each other and add up faster than you think. The exercise changes your brain, so sticking to a healthier eating plan is more manageable and junk food loses its hold over you. From a weight loss perspective, burning calories pales in comparison with the cognitive benefits exercise bestows, transforming you into a better eater.

THE TORTOISE WINS THIS RACE

A slow and steady approach (breaking a big project into manageable pieces) allows you to learn to love the journey so it doesn't seem as if you've sold yourself into weight loss slavery. This isn't white-knuckle lifestyle change, where with every passing day you have an increased desire to stab a badger in the kidney with a salad fork, or one where you can maybe power through for a few weeks or months but are doomed to backslide.

Starving yourself while suffering through sweat sessions to drop a few inches for a high school reunion, then beginning to regain weight the instant you hit the buffet line is not smart. That's losing it *wrong*. Going slowly and steadily means you won't be constantly thinking about being on a diet or engaging in an exercise program; healthy eating and physical fitness will just become part of who you are. No more yoyo weight loss.

Although this book is called *Lose It Right*, we want you to know it doesn't have all the answers. You have an important role to play in adapting this program to your life, personality and physiology. Everyone is different. Overall, it's about following a tolerable pace, and you determine what "tolerable" is.

Be a tortoise instead of a hare. You will reap benefits.

BE THIS

Before proceeding further, you must wrap your brain around this fact: this is not a weight loss book. This is not a "get in shape" book. This is a lifestyle overhaul book.

Deep down, most of us have an idea about what achieves lasting weight loss . . . that healthy-eating-and-exercise thing. What most of us don't know is how to become a person who lives that way. Teaching you how to do this is our focus.

You need to be motivated, and the best way to do that is through understanding what you're in for and *how* to change—not just your body but your mind, your schedule and your reason for being. It's not just about the exercises you engage in and the diet you consume; it's about changing who you are.

It's not a list of actions. It's someone you become.

Don't just do this; be this.

STAGE 1:
LEARN

1

WHY WE'RE FAT, PART 1
— THE WORLD WE LIVE IN

Action is the antidote to despair.

—JOAN BAEZ

To embrace the solution, you must first understand the problem. Hang on to your love handles; this could be painful.

FORKS VERSUS FEET

During the 24-year period between 1976 and 2000 there was more than a doubling of people qualifying as "obese" in the United States; the figure rose from 15 percent to 30.9 percent of the population.[1] Part of this was due to an overall decrease in physical activity (feet). A recent study by Pennington Biomedical Research Center in Louisiana found that in the past 50 years in the US, occupation-related energy expenditure has decreased by approximately 100 calories per day.[2] More important, however, is that caloric *intake* has gone up (forks). A lot. Between 1970 and 2000 the average American increased daily energy intake by 500 calories.[3]

That's a five-to-one ratio of eating more to moving less. These are approximations, of course, but the numbers are damning no matter how you crunch them.

The important question to ask, then, is why are we moving less and eating more?

NO SINGLE CAUSE

We live in what's known as an "obesigenic environment," which is scientist speak for "it makes you fat." Sedentary jobs, busy schedules and easy access to nutritionally compromised yet calorie-packed "food" we don't have to cook is what modern life is all about. There is 24/7 access to highly palatable (junk) food that's hard to resist. Near-constant eating has become so ingrained in our culture that it's difficult to withstand the call of the cookie, the Krispy Kreme or the cheeseburger. As a result, the pounds pack on, and they don't come off easily.

But there's more to it than abundance and inactivity. The truth is, there's no one cause for people being overweight. Some shout, "It's all carbs' fault!" but sorry, that ain't why we're fat. The root causes of overweight and obesity are as diverse as the people carrying those extra pounds. It's only the charlatans who will point out a universal cause and say, "This is why you're fat."

So, what are some of these myriad causes? Let's tackle the environmental issues first.

WORKING OURSELVES TO DEATH

The comedian and philosopher George Carlin once said, "We've learned how to make a living, but not a life. We've added years to life, not life to years."

He had a point. Tell me if this daily routine sounds at all familiar to you: *Get up. Wake kids up. Brush teeth. Wake kids up again. Shower. Wake kids up again,* for real this time! *Preen. Caffeine. "You're going to be late for school!" Breakfast? Are you kidding? Commute hell. Cube hell. Food zoo hell. Commute hell again. Help with homework hell. Dial for pizza. Taxi kids to wherever. Kill brain cells with TV. Not tonight, I have a headache. Repeat.*

If you're like many people, work is slowly killing you. Somewhere in the not too distant past, we went from working to live to living to work. Hours are long and stress is high. We're tethered to smartphones, and everyone wants everything yesterday. Saddled with debts, we still desire more stuff, and the way to get it is more work, more money. If you make enough you can also fund a comfortable retirement, but you might not be around to spend it, because the stress, lack of exercise and massive midsection might make your heart go supernova first.

Talk about messed-up priorities.

People working for companies aren't the only ones who are at risk. As rewarding as homemaking can be, those who stay at home are under more stress than ever before to be super-parents who do everything and do it well. Everyone is overworked and needs a break.

And so it's not just the advent of highly palatable food permeating society that's making people fat, but the fact that most of it is also quick and easy. Since 1955 the amount that Americans have spent eating restaurant food (which includes things such as ordering pizza and hitting the drive-through) has risen from 25 percent of food budgets to 49 percent.[4]

And eating takeout food is on the upswing. It used to be that when people ate outside the home, it was at least a sit-down meal in a restaurant, but by 2006 more than 60 percent of these restaurant meals were to go, being eaten at home, at the office or in the car.[5] And this doesn't take into consideration the massive growth of easy-to-prepare, out-of-a-box processed junk at the grocery store. What started with Swanson TV dinners back in 1953 has exploded into grocery store freezer aisles filled with products from multiple manufacturers all looking to make a buck by making your life easier.

It's become easy to get a high-calorie wallop any time of day with no effort. You can order via phone or Internet, detour a few minutes on your way home through a drive-through or take the family to dinner-tainment at a restaurant that makes eating fun.

Time pressure is what makes all this so appealing.

Work lives are harried; we feel as if we don't have time or energy to put toward planning, shopping for, preparing and cleaning up after proper meals. Instead, you can buy a bucket of Kentucky Fried Grease Chunks and dip the skin in the gravy while watching some mindless TV. The kids aren't going to complain. They'll say, "KFC! Yay!" You'll be a hero. It didn't cost too much more than preparing a meal yourself, you didn't have to shop for groceries or spend time cooking, and cleanup involves cramming stuff into the bucket and throwing the whole lot in the garbage. Cleaning out your arteries is the only hard part.

And don't forget the snacking culture that comes with the modern-day working life. Meetings have doughnuts and cookies, people bring chocolates into the office, and rarely do we pass up an opportunity to eat. Tasty food is always happening, and we partake readily because we're so stressed out and overworked that we *need* an easy source of pleasure.

And so our culture has changed from one that valued food as fuel to one that thinks about food as pleasure.

Time to Rebel

It's time to rebel. In order to live a happy, healthy and hopefully long life, you must find a way to embrace working to live rather than living to work. And this applies to *any* kind of work. There are times the bathroom needs cleaning and the lawn needs mowing and countless other items need to be checked off the endless to-do list. But I'll often de-prioritize these tasks in favor of a bike ride and feel better for it. I'll be *happier*, even though my toilet doesn't smell like a rose garden.

And here's an important fact to keep your personal rebellion on track: working beyond 40 hours a week is shown to cause an *overall* drop in productivity. What this means is that you can actually get more done in 40 hours than in 60.[6]

Work less, live more. Sound easy? This is anything *but* easy, which is why (as with everything) we advise a slow and steady approach to changing your lifestyle. You shouldn't just quit your job and go live on a commune with a bunch of deodorant-optional hippies. However, there are ways you can gradually decrease the time you're run ragged with an endless pile of work (any kind of work), which will in turn decrease your overall stress and make you better able to buy your food from the grocery store and prepare it yourself (as well as find time to exercise).

Once upon a time, I had a choice to make. I had the opportunity to make a good deal more money than I earn right now. The catch? A life-sucking career path. I talked it over with my wife, who was pushing for the "screw that life" option, and I said screw that life. She did too. She could have signed on for crazy hours in her own career, but she chose not to. We'd started a family and wanted to be around to be parents—healthy parents—and have some fun with life.

Maybe our approach can work for you. Maybe you can focus less on expensive toys and more on fun outside. Maybe you can lower your standards, stop trying to keep up with the Joneses and work fewer hours. Just as with weight loss, it won't happen quickly or easily, but maybe you'll find a way to prioritize health. We'll share more details on how to make this happen in Stage II, Prepare.

ALL STRESSED OUT AND NOTHING TO EAT

So, convenient food that someone else cooks alleviates some of the pressure of a busy, often chaotic life. Okay. But what about using highly palatable food to alleviate stress? The so-called emotional eating?

As already examined, work contributes to high stress levels, but it goes beyond an overbearing boss, malicious co-workers and semi-literate clients.

It's no surprise that emotional trauma can lead to a search for comfort. For some, that comfort comes in the form of drugs, for others it's alcohol. Some seek solace in self-destructive sexual behaviors, and some choose food to fill the void created by negative life experiences. These experiences can be from childhood, the more recent past or just from getting yelled at by your boss at your 10 a.m. "team" meeting.

And sometimes emotional eating isn't caused by trauma at all; it's just a result of the world you grew up in.

"When I was upset as a child my mother would start making a chocolate cake that I called the 'crisis cake,'" television reporter Leeza Gibbons told me. "It was the process of making the cake with my mother that was very therapeutic. I'd sit on the counter and we'd make it together and talk about whatever was bothering me, and by the time the cake was ready my issue was resolved. The problem was, we still ate the cake."

"If you were upset, Mom would make food," Jen McKinnon, a 33-year-old mother of four in Calgary, told me. "Or if you were celebrating, it was about food too. Everything growing up was about food." It took until adulthood for McKinnon to break with this conditioning. For her, exercise was the key component in doing so.

Love and attention are great ways to deal with stress, but food doesn't need to be part of the equation. In Gibbons's example, she could have had all the benefits of Mom Therapy during a walk or a knitting session.

But Gibbons and McKinnon are hardly alone. Stress is on the rise worldwide. In Britain, this is evidenced by the record profits being hauled in by producers of tasty snacks. They've seen a massive annual increase in sales of premium treats (mostly chocolate). Regardless of cost or health consequences, people reported that gratifying their taste buds was a priority; they considered it "me time."[7]

In 1991, Harvard University psychologists determined that people who binge eat are "motivated by a desire to escape from self-awareness." Such people are often sensitive to the perceived demands of others and have unflattering views of themselves. This emotional distress, which can include anxiety and depression, causes them to focus on the immediate gratification obtained via food to temporarily escape from negative thoughts.[8]

"People's stress is increasing," says Leigh Gibson, a professor of biopsychology at the University of Roehampton in London. "Time seems to be a much harder commodity to have enough of these days. I fear that technology has contributed to this." Then we half-joked over how we were stressed about our repeated email pings during our conversation. We felt the compulsion to check those emails.

Tell Me about Your Childhood

Wendy Williams is a syndicated talk-show host with four million viewers daily. Successful, right? But being ridiculed as the overweight one in the family once drove her into a vicious circle of comfort eating, as well as other destructive behaviors such as bingeing and purging, taking diets pills and downing mega-doses of laxatives.

"My mother would bring cookies home for my brother and I'd bribe him to give me some of them," Wendy told me. "Once I got my driver's license I could go to McDonald's and eat a couple of McRibs and then go home for dinner and act like it never happened."

I'm familiar with the impulse. Growing up I was both unathletic and weird, so I didn't have many friends. My weekends comprised shoveling in junk food like a crocodile with a mouthful of wildebeest, rotting my brain with TV and dreading Monday. This habit of eating crap continued well into my 20s, when I discovered exercise (prompted by seeing what I now use as a "before" picture). Exercise was the catalyst for changing my diet.

But I still struggle. I know that after a rough day I'll hit the liquor store instead of the bike path. It takes mental gymnastics to think my way toward the right decision and resist ordering pizza or scarfing down a box of chocolate chip cookies because I don't feel like cooking. I don't always succeed.

"By eating sweet foods you're able to activate a number of brain systems that relieve stress and improve mood," Gibson told me. "You can demonstrate that it improves tolerance for pain, for example." The feelings are immediate but transient, lasting only a few minutes, he said. And what's worse, you may experience guilt afterward for having eaten junk food, which wipes out the uplifting effects even more quickly.

Who Is at Risk?

"There is substantial evidence that women are more likely to express comfort eating than men," Gibson said. "Women are also more likely to suffer depression than men."

He spoke of a recent study out of San Diego showing that people with higher depression scores had higher chocolate intakes. The connection was more apparent in women. "It was a very strong relationship," he said. "Clearly there is something about being depressed that drives wanting chocolate." It's not curing the depression, though.

And just being poor at dealing with stress puts you at risk as well. "Emotional eaters are not as good at coping with stress," says Gibson. To a certain extent, the more stressed or depressed you are, the more likely you are to seek solace from highly palatable food.

For Wendy Williams, it took the birth of her son 12 years ago to get her to reevaluate her life and become happy with being a big woman. Now she exercises and focuses on clean eating, but she still enjoys indulgences in a healthy way.

I spoke to her the day after Hurricane Sandy made landfall in New York. She was having a "natural-disaster binge day," sharing tasty treats with her family out of the fridge and freezer in case they lost power and things began to spoil.

"We've got cookie dough in the freezer," she told me. "We can't let that go bad!"

Food can still be a source of enjoyment. You can use it to celebrate or even to make light of a bad situation. But you've got to look at how often these things are happening. You've got to ask if you're eating feelings.

THE FOOD ENVIRONMENT

That covers work and stress. Now you know how time pressure (work) and blood pressure (stress) conspire to make us reach for the nearest convenience food. This statement is probably going to result in hate mail, but I put some of the blame for our current addiction to convenience food on men. I can do that because I am one—one who cooks.

Meal Preparation and Misandry

See, women used to stay home and do the grocery shopping and prepare the meals. Then, in the latter half of the 20th century, they entered the workforce in droves and men didn't pick up the slack on the home front. After a day of work it was still somehow the woman's job to take care of housework and meal preparation. With men not doing their share, women looked for a way to ease the burden, and capitalism came to the "rescue." You know, TV dinners, pizza delivery, drive-through windows open 24 hours a day . . .

"There are many more high-calorie foods available now," says Nicole Avena, a research neuroscientist in the fields of diet and addiction at the University of Florida College of Medicine. "They're easy and convenient. There is also the palatability factor. We've seen that foods have become more complicated. The ingredients used contain lots of added fats and sugars, which improve taste, but also brings along lots of calories, which are empty calories. They have little to no nutritional value."

Earlier in this chapter I pointed out that the percentage of American food dollars spent eating out has doubled in the past half century. An absence of grocery shopping and meal preparation has become culturally ingrained in North America. Cooking is a lost art, and the food that other people make for you has too many calories in it, tastes far too good, and the portions are way too big.

Built to Consume

"We have a society built around consumption."

My friend Dr. Yoni Freedhoff, an obesity expert in Ottawa, said that to me. "We don't see it any more clearly than when it comes to food. There is nowhere people can go that junk food is not provided."

Welcome to the modern-day obesigenic environment, where we've gone from scarcity to plenty. Don't get me wrong: plenty is awesome. Beats the hell out of starving to death. But things are out of control. It's more capitalism run amok.

Capitalism, by the way, is also awesome. (Tell your friends to buy this book.) However, there are lines that can be crossed, and some food company executives have gone all Darth Vader on us.

I'm not going to get into some libertarian versus socialist argument about what should or should not be done to rein in food corporations. Plenty of others better qualified than me have debated this subject in many different forums. I'm just going to report on how things are so you know what you're up against and can plan accordingly how to navigate your way through this environment in as healthy a manner as possible. We can bitch and moan about how wrong it all is, but the fact is that things aren't going to change soon, so it's your job to understand the situation and take appropriate action to look after your own health and the health of those you care for.

The Former Big-Food Executive

"Food companies are not focused on making healthy food, they are focused on making profits," said Bruce Bradley, who has held senior marketing positions with companies such as General Mills, Pillsbury and Nabisco. "They want you to eat more. They make money by selling more food."

I suppose that makes sense. It's how they do it that's sinister.

"The way they get us to buy more food is by making it irresistible," Bradley told me. They use lots of sugar, fat and salt to get you eating more. As you'll discover in chapter 2, that's bad.

And a lot of the time, they'll pretend these products are healthy by using words like "whole grains," Bradley said, but they are still full of unhealthy ingredients. "When you're making processed foods you use ingredients that allow a product to stay on the shelf for a year or two and still taste good."

I think I just lost my appetite.

Protecting Themselves with Profits

"Government lobbying is one of the biggest things the food industry does to protect and grow its profits," Bradley said. "It's about setting the rules of the game as loose as possible."

Anyone with a business degree knows that the goal of any corporation is to maximize shareholder value. They don't care about *you* unless caring about you somehow makes them more money. And in most cases it's not caring about you that increases profits. And so the industry lobbies those who should protect us to keep regulations lax.

This isn't a conspiracy theory. I don't believe the moon landings were faked, or that aliens abduct people out of trailer parks and probe them, or that the Kardashian clan is the result of an unholy union between the Loch Ness Monster and a rabid sasquatch. Actually, I'm on the fence about that last one.

Although I'm a skeptic, I accept that this is the reality of our profit-driven economy, and in weight loss territory it's your enemy. To live healthfully in this day and age, you need to learn how to navigate the influence of food corporations and restaurants because the government isn't going to do it for you.

Where I live, Health Canada is the "federal department responsible for helping Canadians maintain and improve their health."[9] Several years ago, Dr. Freedhoff was involved in consultations with Health Canada on the development of the new food guide. He asserts that the department is not interested in anything that makes Canadians more aware of caloric intake.

"I think it's insane that the food guide provides zero guidance on calories," he told me. "We've had a number of bills presented to government to put calories on restaurant menus, and they always get struck down. I know that the food industry has opposed calorie labeling. They ultimately oppose anything that affects sales."

The situation is no different in the United States. The Academy of Nutrition and Dietetics (formerly the American Dietetic Association) is funded by myriad food companies such as Coca-Cola, PepsiCo and Kellogg's,[10] and the National Restaurant Association is a strategic partner to promote the United States Department of Agriculture's (USDA) "MyPlate" (which replaced the "food pyramid" in 2011). As a reminder, restaurants, like food corporations, are also vested in repeat business, which means making food taste great, which translates to "irresistible and high in calories." Having an association whose raison d'être is to promote the interests of restaurants partner with the USDA on guidelines for how Americans should eat is ludicrous. "We are restaurants' champion" is right there on the About Us page of the NRA website.[11] Oh, wait. Not *that* NRA. This NRA's ammunition is shaped more like cheese sticks.

Can open. Worms everywhere.

The dining-out NRA has four areas that they focus on for their members, and the first one is about profitability. The fourth one mentions social responsibility, but they're talking about environmental sustainability and charity work, not doing what's right for the health of the nation's citizens. There's a mention of increasing consumer awareness about nutritional information, but this is because they're interested in "building and sustaining positive public opinion and a favorable political environment."[12] And so they flog MyPlate. You scratch my back . . .

And, of course, right below the public opinion/political environment part they get into "helping grow revenues" and "increase profitability . . ."

Too bad that government agriculture subsidies aren't in line with supporting what's on MyPlate. A 2012 release from the US Public Interest Research Group determined that government subsidization of junk-food additives pays for 21 Twinkies per taxpayer per year, but those same taxpayers only get half an apple paid for.[13] If you want apples, you must pay for them yourself, but here, have some junk food.

According to Bruce Bradley, consumers don't stand a chance of knowing what's in their food. All the government lobbying, misinformation and backroom collaboration make it difficult to reach a sound judgment about what to eat.

And I've barely scratched the surface.

The Broader Impact

Charlene Elliot is an associate professor of food marketing at the University of Calgary. She explained how the reach of food companies with child-centric products is growing. It used to be limited to the cereal aisle, but now there is a grocery-store-wide heap of food about as "real" as Milli Vanilli.

The focus is on artificiality. "It's shaped like bugs, stars and princesses," Elliot said. "It glows in the dark. You can tattoo your tongue with a fruit roll-up. Hannah Montana's face is right there on your waffles." It's all about upping the fun factor of food. Unfortunately, "there's a direct link between eating for fun, sport or entertainment and obesity," Elliot said.

And it doesn't stop there. "The food industry has come up with a line of 'better for you' products," she continued. "We did an analysis comparing them with the regular products, and while they were somewhat better for you, they were certainly not good for you." That's a distinction worth paying attention to. This "nutritionism" reduces food to its component parts, where marshmallow pebbles are "healthy" because they have vitamin D added. A protein bar is just another kind of chocolate bar, but it's got protein, so it must be awesome, right? Cover a granola bar in chocolate and caramel goo and the granola is still supposed to make it a healthy choice.

I'll Take That Sugar and Fat to Go, Please

Elliot goes on to explain that there's been a big move toward portable food. "Snack sizes" and "to go" items are heavily marketed these days. It's as though the food companies are telling us that no matter where we go, we must have conveniently packaged food to take with us. Clearly, we shouldn't be allowed to stop eating for more than a few minutes at a time.

Gee . . . bananas, oranges and apples aren't portable at all. You need some sugar-fat concoction in a plastic package instead.

I'm starting to think auto manufacturers are in on it. My family has a Toyota minivan. It seats seven, but it has 17 cup holders! That's more than two and a half cup holders *per passenger*. Is Toyota expecting me to host a frat party in there?

And let's not even get started on the whole topic of who gets to decide what a "serving size" is. Grab a to-go bag of potato chips in the impulse aisle at the grocery store checkout and it will say a serving is about 150 calories. That doesn't sound so bad, right? Not until you do the math and note that there are two or three of those servings in that little bag, and you were fully intending to eat that whole thing. If you're not paying close attention, it's easier to consume far more calories than you'd intended. And the food companies know that. The serving size list in the nutritional information is not a reflection of how much the typical consumer eats. Not even close.

Gimme More

In North America, we love a bargain.

"There is a 'good deal' mentality," said Lisa Young, a registered dietitian, adjunct professor at New York University and an expert in portion sizes. "People will absolutely go to restaurants with larger portion sizes. We think that we need Godzilla portions to be satiated."

We also have a clean plate mentality. "Even if you don't clean your plate, you're still eating a lot. There's also the doggie bag mentality." If you resist temptation and only eat half your meal, the rest of that high-calorie dinner is going to get eaten at some point or another.

Young explains that restaurant food has high caloric density, and when it's combined with the large portion sizes, the total amount of calories in the typical restaurant meal is massive. Remember, half of American food dollars are spent eating out. It's a major contributor to the obesity epidemic.

We can thank the food industry's competitive environment for some of this, says Young. Those larger portion sizes "allow them to charge more," she says. "[A restaurant] can add five cents' worth of food and charge 25 cents more for it." That's a good profit margin, and, as Bruce Bradley said, the food business is all about profit.

So just how much larger are those portions? According to the Centers for Disease Control, since 1950 restaurant meals have increased by a shocking 400 percent! Seven-ounce sodas became 42 ounces. Four-ounce burgers transformed into 12 ounces. Two-and-a-half-ounce orders of fries grew to almost seven ounces.[14]

This offers some explanation about why we're so much heavier now than we were then.

Designed to Be Irresistible?

During my chat with Bruce Bradley, I asked him if food companies purposely try to make food irresistible.

"It's not so direct," he said. "There is no evil backroom meeting. It's more of a perspective where you start drinking the Kool-Aid." He explained that it's about making delicious food and seeing if people come back and eat more. "When you measure it like that it seems innocent, but in the big picture it's more nefarious. The impact adds up over many products."

It seems I'm not the only one wondering about this issue. In 2005 reporters from the *Chicago Tribune* did a multi-piece exposé of Kraft's efforts to boost sales of products like the Oreo cookie. This is from the article: "Kraft said it does not conduct research 'aimed at creating consumer dependency upon any of our products.' At the same time, internal memos show the company has a history of sharing brain-research expertise with scientists from its corporate sibling, cigarette-maker Philip Morris."[15]

Wait a minute. *Kraft shared brain-research expertise with a cigarette company?*

The piece reported that they shared government lobbyists too.

A 2006 follow-up piece, also in the *Chicago Tribune*, reported that "Kraft and Philip Morris scientists traded ideas for studying the fine details of how the brain processes tastes and smells. A 1997 planning memo proposed investing in 'neuroimaging,' or brain scans, and research on sensory neuroreceptors, which are sites on brain cells that process smells and tastes."[16]

The article alleged that at the time, both Philip Morris and Kraft were under the same parent company, the Altria Group. Miller Brewing was part of the same family, and a 1998 memo suggested that the three companies should collaborate on how to engineer products that would influence a customer's mood or sense of fullness.[17]

Purveyors of booze, smokes and Oreos working together to raise profits via mutually beneficial brain

Is Food Addictive?

Food can be compelling as hell, but addictive? Not according to a 2012 study in *Nature Reviews*. The authors concluded that although highly palatable food may have addictive-like properties, it does not meet all the criteria of an addictive substance. "The vast majority of overweight individuals have not shown a convincing behavioral or neurobiological profile that resembles addiction," the authors wrote.[18]

Despite efforts by some to have food addiction included, the fifth edition of the *Diagnostic and Statistical Manual of Mental Disorders* (DSM) did not classify "food" as an addiction. According to Nicole Avena, even though highly palatable food affects the same brain mechanisms that addictive drugs do, there is not enough evidence to warrant a full psychiatric diagnosis for food addiction. "There are a lot of differences between food and drugs," she said.

"It's a matter of degree and vulnerability," said Carolyn Davis, a professor at York University in Toronto specializing in the psychobiology of obesity. "Regular drinkers aren't necessarily addicts; they aren't dependent. When it comes to food, I think it's a small population that is truly addicted." Davis said she was struggling to separate food addiction from an extreme form of binge-eating disorder, which is in the DSM. "'Food addiction' isn't a good term," she said.

research. Right about now you should be making a reference to sacramental excrement.

Eating Outside the Box

Are food corporations evil?

After reading this chapter, do you now imagine Satan sitting at his desk down in Hell shuffling papers as he reads about the despicable deeds of some food company executives, and wondering how to assign the appropriate level of damnation when they show up on his infernal doorstep? "What's the right kind of eternal torment for the guy who said marshmallow pebbles are healthy?" he might ask himself. "How far do I stick my pitchfork up the keester of the one who wanted to make cookies as addictive as cigarettes?"

Evil or not is a question for moral philosophers. I will, however, point out that consumers helped create the situation. It's supply and demand. The food companies are, to a large degree, giving us what we want. Companies that focus on what we need to sustain health don't always last long, because, as we've established, most humans are driven by a desire for pleasure, not health, when it comes to eating.

Morality aside, I'm here to tell you to avoid their wares.

In my interview with Leigh Gibson, he compared the current food environment to an arms race: food corporations are battling over your money, and they're investing in research and development to create the best weapons for blowing away your taste buds. So how do you find peace in this cold cereal war? How do you navigate the obesigenic environment to thrive, be healthy and lean? Answer: you don't.

I mean, you don't navigate it. You reject it. Most of the time you just have to stay away.

Freedhoff, Elliot, Avena and Bradley all agree: the trick is just not to eat as many processed foods. You can't believe the marketing and health claims that the food industry wants you to swallow (as much as they want you to swallow their food products). They're trying to get you to believe that a wide variety of junk food is a healthy choice. It's not healthy. Don't believe them.

So understand that junk food isn't healthy, and armed with that knowledge do your best to make it an occasional indulgence instead of a staple. Plan indulgences for when you *want* them, and pick something that you'll enjoy to treat yourself. Don't fall for the health-washing.

Yes, you can still eat junk food sometimes. It's a treat, and we all deserve occasional decadence. The goal here is to make you realize the need to live by that word "occasional."

"Stick with the unprocessed fare," Charlene Elliot says. "The idea of fun with food is not healthy."

"I don't think these foods should be outlawed," Bruce Bradley adds. "But they shouldn't be disguised as health foods."

Even though she has a book that helps people control portions and that offers advice for limiting caloric intake while eating out, Lisa Young admits the safest bet is to stay home. "At home you're in control of the food you're eating, but in a restaurant you really have no control over what's being served in terms of calories."

If you want to be successful at sustained weight loss, you must take control of your food preparation. It doesn't need to be complicated or fancy, but meals made at home using fresh ingredients are the only solution.

The End of Overeating

If you want to delve further into the mysteries of the food industry, I (partially) recommend Dr. David Kessler's *The End of Overeating*. I write "partially" because Kessler's theory of "Food Rehab" is wrong for recommending a zero tolerance eating strategy (more on this in chapter 9), but the book does offer good information on the massive amount of calories packed into foods in ways you wouldn't imagine. Specifically, there are useful explanations about how extra calories are piled into restaurant food to make it taste extra yummy. Read it and you'll understand why we recommend that you go back to those 1955 levels of food dollars spent on eating out.

If you read Dr. Kessler's book, you may never eat fast food again.

2

WHY WE'RE FAT, PART 2
— THE SCIENCE OF SIZE

You must unlearn what you have learned.

—YODA, *The Empire Strikes Back*

As we learned in chapter 1, obesity is a multi-factorial condition. That means it has more causes than *Cosmo* has freaky sex tips.

In the simplest sense, however, obesity has just *one* cause: consistent positive energy balance. In English, this means taking in more calories than you burn. But before we get into that, I have to explain why calories matter.

WEIGHT LOSS MATH

It's really simple. If you have a caloric deficit, you lose weight. If calories are positive, you gain weight (we'll get into making weight loss about *fat loss* later). Energy balance is a direct representation of the first law of thermodynamics, the one that says energy can neither be created nor destroyed. We're not talking about a hypothesis here, or even a theory, but a physical LAW OF THE UNIVERSE. Ever hear of the law of gravity? A law is something scientists are so damn sure of that there's no disputing it. You can't deny the first law of thermodynamics any more than you can deny the fact that if you jump out of a high-flying airplane without a parachute, gravity will not be your friend. (Note to fans of *The Secret*: the "Law of Attraction" is not a real scientific law.)

And yes, I do know there are best-selling authors who question this law. They present themselves as "controversial." They assert that years of accepted science are wrong. Let me ask you a question: the next time you get into an airplane, would you rather it was designed, built and tested in a scientifically proven manner, or in a controversial one?

I thought so.

Excess fat can't be blamed on insulin, carbohydrates or the Loch Ness Monster. Gaining body fat comes from taking in more calories than you burn. Anyone who can prove otherwise will surely win a Nobel Prize in physics for disproving the first law of thermodynamics. I am unaware of that particular Nobel having been awarded.

Back on planet Earth, the link between weight loss and calories has been proven myriad times.

Rudolph Leibel et al. conducted a carefully controlled study in 1992, which was published in the *American Journal of Clinical Nutrition* and asserted that "variations in fat intake from 0% to 70% of total energy under conditions of equal energy intake produced no significant changes in body weight over periods of observation averaging 33 d [days]." In language that we can all understand: Leibel's study put participants on balanced energy diets: they controlled to ensure that the participants took in the same number of calories as they burned over a 33-day period. The participants got a varied range of overall fat content, from 0 percent to 70 percent, but everyone's weight stayed the same, once again proving the first law of thermodynamics.[1]

Why did the participants' weight stay the same? Because they were on maintenance-level calories. It does not matter what percentage of protein, carbohydrates or fat you consume in the grander scheme of weight loss and gain. It's all the simple formula of calories in minus calories out. Obesity researchers Alain Golay and Elisabetta Bobbioni, in their 1997 article "The Role of Dietary Fat in Obesity," agree: "fat is almost exclusively used or stored in response to day-to-day fluctuations in energy balance."[2]

In 2004 nutrition professors Andrea Buchholz and Dale Schoeller looked at the published data to answer the question, is a calorie a calorie? The results were published in the *American Journal of Clinical Nutrition*.

The authors conducted a thorough metabolic analysis of the effects of diets that varied in fat, protein and carbohydrates and made this assertion: "We conclude that a calorie is a calorie. From a purely thermodynamic point of view, this is clear because the human body or, indeed, any living organism cannot create or destroy energy but can only convert energy from one form to another."[3]

Beyond this, there is so much research that proves the whole calories-in vs. calories-out rule[4] that any arguments claiming that weight loss is something other than an energy balance issue are as real as professional wrestling. What's more, I've interviewed a number of the world's top obesity researchers, and for every one it's a "well, duh!" that weight loss is calories in versus calories out, regardless of the type of calories.

If you eat 2,000 calories of chicken wings and butter-fried pork rinds a day yet burn 2,500 calories a day, you will lose weight. You will also be one unhealthy bugger.

If you eat 3,000 calories of spinach, carrots and egg whites a day yet burn 2,500 calories a day, you will gain weight. Harsh, but true.

The Twinkie Diet

Is this sinking in? Although it didn't qualify as an official study, Mark Haub's experiment bears consideration. Haub is a nutrition professor at Kansas State University, although you may know him better as "Twinkie Guy." In 2010, Twinkie Guy proved he could lose weight living mostly on Twinkies, Doritos, Oreos and other treats just by consuming fewer calories than he burned. He lost 27 pounds in two months, though I imagine that due to the low satiety factor and high reward value of the food, he must have felt he was starving the entire time. He didn't do the experiment to endorse a junk food weight loss program but to prove a point: calories are all that matter to weight loss.

As we'll show, it's far easier to sustain a lower caloric intake when food is healthy than when it's sugary-fatty-salty crap. Remember that sustainable weight loss is about finding a healthy way to have a reasonable caloric deficit while losing weight and then finding a healthy way to sustain caloric balance when you achieve your target weight.

BEYOND THE NUMBERS

In chapter 1, and at the beginning of this chapter, I mentioned that a positive energy balance (taking in more calories than you need) has multiple causes. Let's get graphic and check out some of them.

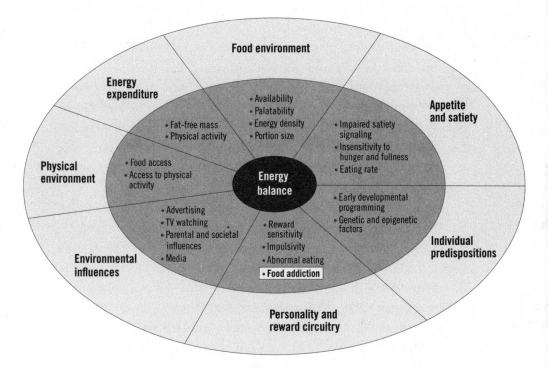

Mediators of Energy Balance and Body Weight

This figure is taken from a 2012 article by University of Cambridge researchers published in *Nature Reviews*.[5] It lists the wide variety of factors that contribute to overweight and obesity. Yup, there are a lot of them. For now let's look at one you *can't* change.

Genetics and the Art of Sucking It Up

Heredity is not destiny.

If you saw my parents in their swimsuits you'd understand that I'm not genetically programmed for leanness. (And now I'm out of their wills.)

That being said, some of us are naturally inclined to be heavier than others. However, recall the stat that we threw out at the beginning of the previous chapter, the one about the doubling of obesity rates in the United States in only 24 years. The genetics of humanity do not change so quickly; the rapid rise must be coming from those environmental causes we discussed. However, the way in which individuals react to this new environment can be genetic. It can also be *epigenetic*: the environment modifies the way your genes are expressed. Creepy.

Here's the thing. Your genes are what they are. You can't change them. There's far more that we *don't* know about the genetic causes of obesity than we do, so it doesn't make sense to do a massive deconstruction of the various genes that may or may not make you more susceptible to weight gain. This is one of those things that fall under the heading "Suck It Up."

Some people have to work harder than others to be fit and healthy, but it's important to know that even for those of us genetically programmed to be overweight, hard work can *get 'er done*. Need proof? Let's look at the Pima Indians. Several studies have compared a group of Pima in Arizona with Pima in a remote area of Mexico. The two groups have a shared genetic background programmed by their specific evolutionary circumstances to gain weight easily so they could live through frequent famines, but their circumstances are not at all alike. The Arizona Pima have a lifestyle that requires far less manual labor and provides access to ample high-calorie foods. As a result, the Arizona tribe has one of the highest rates of obesity and type 2 diabetes in the world. By contrast, women in the Mexican Pima tribe are just barely overweight on average, and most men are in the normal weight range.[6]

Unlike in Arizona, Mexican Pima live a Spartan existence with much physical activity and moderate caloric intake. Even though they are genetically programmed to be overweight, their lifestyle has created a different outcome. Granted, that lifestyle is one of poverty, but from a genetic perspective it provides proof that no one is destined to be fat. Some people just have to work harder at controlling their weight. The unlucky ones have to work exceptionally hard.

You may have been screwed in the genetic lottery, but I'm about to go all tough love on you. You've got to play the hand you're dealt. There is not one damn thing you can do about your DNA, so it, more than anything else, is something you're just going to have to live with. You may not be destined to look like a fitness model—few of us are—but you *can* improve. You can work with what you've got.

As the old US Army slogan said, Be all you can be.

YOUR BRAIN ON FOOD

Still friends after that tough love bit? Great. Let's move on to learning about how your brain reacts to the food you eat and how that affects your weight and your health.

Reward Systems Run Amok

Have you seen *Trainspotting*, that movie about heroin addiction? It's a serious bummer and I don't recommend it.

There's a scene in which a woman injects the drug for the first time and she says . . . well, I can't write what she says because I'm trying to keep things PG. Anyway, she suggests that heroin is way better than sex. I'd never touch heroin, so I can't weigh in on the debate, but it does make me wonder what kind of lame lovers she's had.

Why all this talk of heroin? Because although the degree is far less, highly palatable food hijacks your brain's reward system in the same manner.[7]

Why We Like What We Like

Think of an apple. Imagine taking a big bite. Even if you *love* apples, you can't imagine eating six of them at once, right? Because no matter how good they are, it's not as though your mouth just had an orgasm, is it?

Crème brûlée, though? Or cookie dough ice cream? Or "Mmmm . . . I love Turtles"? Total mouthgasm.

Unlike a real orgasm, however, junk food doesn't offer much of an afterglow. Plowing through half a pizza or a box of chocolates may make you feel good for a few minutes, but that feeling doesn't stick around for the rest of the day. A sexual romp can keep you sated for a long time, but junk food begets more junk food: you keep eating well beyond the point of bodily energy requirements, losing track of how much you ate and being unable to tell whether you're still hungry. Why do you do this? Because the reward is *outstanding*. Before you know it, the compulsion grows, and you need ever more sugar, salt and fat to quench the desire for the next mouthgasm.

I'm going to stop writing that word now, okay?

Here's the thing: evolution programmed us to like certain flavors. One of the reasons we like sweetness is that it represents nutrition. A piece of fruit is at its nutritional peak when it's at its sweetest. For the millennia of human evolution, seeking out sweetness was good—until technology started messing with things and making nutritionally vacant yet calorically dense hyper-flavored sugar-fat combination treats like hot fudge sundaes. What's more, such foods are soft rather than crunchy, allowing for a fast ingestion that generates an immediate sense of pleasure. It seems similar to the difference between smoking heroin and injecting it.

Have you ever had a perfectly ripe mango? It's one of the most amazing-tasting *natural* foods on the planet. One mango has about 130 calories. How many can you eat? I've tried to eat more than one in a sitting, but halfway through the second I didn't want any more. Something in my brain shuts down so a second one doesn't seem that appealing, no matter how good the first one tasted.

Compare that with a high-sugar/high-fat restaurant dessert such as the Keg's carrot cake à la mode. It has 2,344 calories. That's *18 times* as many calories as a mango. I know I would eat the whole thing and then lick the plate clean; the flavor is so overwhelming that all appetite control is lost. (Then I'd have to do a full marathon's worth of running to burn it off. Think on that math.)

So what the hell is going on here? It's neurochemistry. Sugar, fat and salt all create a chemical cascade in your brain, an intricate interaction of hormones, neurotransmitters, endorphins, satiety signals and reward sensations. Mangos are a simple taste of natural sweetness—delicious, yes, but we get bored with it quickly. Processed treats, on the other hand, amplify and combine flavors to create an overwhelming taste sensation that's hard to get tired of. And some people have it worse than others. These poor folk are more "reward sensitive" than the average Joe, and they crave the fix that drugs, alcohol or highly palatable (extra-yummy) food gives them more intensely. Others are what we call "super tasters," experiencing greater taste intensities, both positive and negative. They're more likely to love sweet foods, for example, and hate the bitterness of vegetables.

To get all science-y on you for a minute, what we're talking about here is basic operant conditioning psychology related to the stimulus-response model of behavior change. If a stimulus (such as putting a chocolate bar into your mouth) elicits a positive response (such as thinking, *Whoa, Mama, that tastes good*), the stimulus behavior is reinforced and you seek out that rewarding feeling again and again. It works the other way as well, where a bad taste is seen as punishment, causing you to avoid foods you don't like.

Trying to Love the Green Stuff

Broccoli is so good for you. I wish I liked it.

Blarf. Hate the stuff. I've tried. Can't do it.

There are, however, other green vegetables I have managed to develop a taste for, but it took effort. You know what *doesn't* take effort? Liking cherry pie with vanilla ice cream.[8] And that type of "like" goes way beyond "developing a taste." It's not the same with vegetables, where I can say, "Yeah, this tastes okay. I'll eat it because I know it promotes satiety and is good for me." With a yummy dessert, or cheeseburgers, chicken wings, pizza, chocolate, potato chips, etcetera, it's, *OMG, so good that I can't restrain myself—must have more!*

When I'm faced with such a dessert, it takes an effort of will not to eat it in the first place,[9] because my brain has been conditioned to know it's an instantaneous source of massive pleasure.[10] And if I start eating it, it's hard to stop.[11]

With the veggies, however, it's as if I have to force myself to finish them.

Right now, you're all like, "Well, duh. One tastes so-so and the other tastes amazing." Yes, that is correct. And how these differing tastes affect your brain and cause weight gain is what we're about to get into. It's more complex than yummy versus bitter.

What you eat isn't just about how it tastes. Yes, we've just learned that there is a psychological aspect of "positive reinforcement,"[12] and that this works in reverse as well, where bad-tasting foods are avoided. Beyond this, however, there are also metabolic, endocrine and genetic factors at play.[13] Interestingly, though, it still boils down to the way highly palatable food makes you feel.

What's Going On in There?

It's all about the hippopotamus.

Wait, what? Oh, sorry. *Hypothalamus*. My co-author Margaret insists it's the hypothalamus, and she would know, because of the PhD in neuro-science psychology something something. This is where it is in your brain:

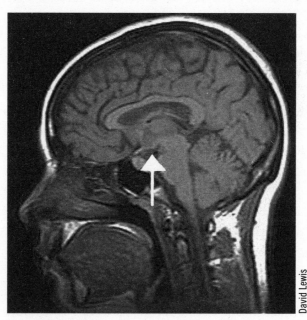

What my co-author looks like without all that hair, skin and skull getting in the way.

There is much recent research about the metabolic and neural feedback signals that are responsible for our desire to eat.[14] Many of these are generated in the hypothalamus, which is like a thermostat for your body. It regulates internal temperature, hunger, thirst and sleep cycles.

So far, so good. If hunger were just a matter of hypothalamic inputs, the brain could hypothetically adjust our appetites to keep our bodies in a healthy weight range; it could stop us from eating when we'd had enough to meet our daily energy requirements.

But that ain't happening.

Our ability to regulate food intake "cannot withstand the strong environmental pressures in most individuals," said Hans-Rudolf Berthoud, neurobiology of nutrition professor at the Pennington Biomedical Research Center in Louisiana. "Our brain is designed to strike a balance," Nicole Avena told me. "But our brain can sense if we're deficient in nutrients. It's possible to be overfed but undernourished." At least, it's been possible in the past century. Junk food provides a lot of calories but little nourishment. For most of human history we didn't have this problem; things are now out of balance. "And the brain is still seeking out those essential nutrients, so it sends out more hunger signals to get them. There is a cognitive element to getting the vitamins and nutrients we need."

Runaway food consumption is a breakdown between two systems that drive eating. One is physiological, called *homeostatic hunger*.[15] It regulates your body's need for sufficient calories to maintain homeostasis.[16] In less scientific terms, it's about fueling your daily energy requirements, and not much else.

The other system is psychological, called *hedonic hunger*. Think of the word *hedonism*. It's all about the pleasure, baby.

Physiological hunger—the kind that keeps weight "normal"—is guided by signals sent from the gut, blood and hypothalamus sensing levels of glucose and amino and fatty acids.[17] If you are experiencing this type of hunger because your body *needs* food, just about anything is going to taste good.

I remember being out for a run once and "bonking," which is a runner's term for, *Oh God need food now feel wretched can't run without food please feed me.* I made it back to my car ready to eat the steering wheel and found a prehistoric granola bar that my wife had left in the glove box. I don't dig granola bars, especially ones whose best-before date is from around the time a baby Justin Bieber burst out of an alien torso, but I wolfed that sucker down as if it was the antidote to fast-acting poison, and it was scrumptious. (Bonking, by the way, is not "working up an appetite." It's low blood sugar remedied with minimal calories.)

On the other side of the equation, psychological hunger—eating for pleasure—arises from a chain of events that start in the middle of the brain, and that bitchin' vibe you get from eating something sweet and fatty hits those same reward paths as drugs, alcohol, gambling and even sex.[18] This is about cravings. You don't *need* to eat this tasty food, but you *want* it.

You want it bad. Even though you know it makes you gain weight. Even though you know it's not good for you. The reason you want it has to do with . . .

Primary Rewards

A "reward" is a stimulus that alters and reinforces behavior.[19] The reward system is nature's way of making sure we don't die.

Here are some examples of primary rewards:

Examples of rewarding behavior	Reward generated
When this thing between my legs touches the thing between that other person's legs, it *feels really good.*	Continuation of the species.
When my mouth feels as if it's been sandpapered with the Gobi desert, a big glass of water *feels really good.*	Not dying of thirst.
When I've been awake and working for days on end, falling asleep even on a pile of rocks *feels really good.*	Prevention of sleep-deprivation psychosis and eventual death.
When I've eaten a lot of food and things work their way southward, going to the bathroom *feels really good.*	Not exploding and blowing partially digested food all over creation like something out of a Monty Python movie.

Okay, sorry about that last image, but you get the idea. Eating is a rewarding behavior that nature programmed into us so we'll be compelled to seek food and therefore not die. Not dying so you can live long enough to do that rewarding touching-of-things-between-the-legs stuff is what evolution via natural selection is about.

The Prime Suspect

There really isn't any doubt about what causes overeating. This sucker is *guilty*.

It's called the *mesolimbic dopamine reward pathway*. When we engage in behavior that enhances survival (fornicating, eating, sleeping, not exploding) this neural pathway is activated.[20] Dopamine is fired from within the limbic system, which resides deep within the brain. Specifically, dopamine comes from the ventral tegmental area and into the nucleus accumbens.

I thought those were big words too. Let's just refer to it as the "hedonic hot spot."[21]

Unfortunately, not all rewarding behaviors have value in prolonging life. Some of them are downright counter to survival, like the unnaturally rewarding effects of drugs, alcohol and overeating highly palatable food.

The Survival Mechanism

Here's the problem, which is also the explanation.

Even with an awful diet, you can live long enough to procreate. These days, vegetables are great for promoting a healthy body weight. They offer a large volume of food for a low number of calories, they contain fiber, which also makes them more satiating, and they take a lot of chewing, which slows the eating process. They're also not the tastiest things around, which ensures that you tire of eating them before you overconsume. In the current food environment, vegetables are your friends when it comes to keeping weight down, not to mention all the nutritional and cancer-fighting benefits they have.

Cavemen and women didn't care about any of that. Cancer? What the hell is that? These guys were lucky to live to 30, and they wanted as many calories as they could get, because starvation was Enemy Number One, even more so than the saber-toothed murder beast. Starvation is still an issue; it has killed more people throughout human history than anything else.

I shall repeat: *Starvation has killed more people throughout human history than anything else.* Gives you some perspective, doesn't it?

Back to the point at hand. "The energy density in fat and sugar is really high," Eric Stice, an eating specialist and senior scientist at the Oregon Research Institute, told me. "So if we find Brussels sprouts alongside sugar beets, we will choose the beets because our body wants more energy-dense foods. It was a survival mechanism."

Something low calorie, like spinach, didn't do nearly as much to enhance a troglodyte's chances of survival as something sweet or fatty did, because of the energy difference. People living on the brink of starvation were programmed via natural selection to cram in as many calories as possible, which caused them to seek out sweet fruits and fatty meats. And if you mix sweet and fatty together, watch out. That's why chocolate—which contains both sugar and fat—has such a high reinforcement value.[22]

This sense of pleasure is innate. We don't need to learn to like it. It's why I was able to watch my son plow through a big piece of chocolate cake on his first birthday with undisguised glee on his face. I mean, what I could see of his face through the layers of frosting.

Going against Gut Instinct

Time for a reality check: your body has no wisdom when it comes to food.

Some alternative practitioners speak of the "wisdom of the body," and hold that humans have an inherent system designed to seek out only the nutrients we need.

Did anyone else just hear a flock of ducks go by? *Quack, quack, quack . . .*

If this was the case, we'd have a kale shortage and childhood obesity would not exist. The only things the body—and brain—respond to immediately are sugar, fat and salt. This is because each of these compounds produces an immediate signal to the brain, telling it that they hold value: energy to allow for movement (like hunting for more food and procreating) and to build up fat stores to survive the next famine.

Salt, of course, is an exception in that it doesn't contain calories, but it is nevertheless critical to survival.[23] It's important for brain development, and the salt that's sweated from our bodies also needs replacing. Food companies have used it liberally to make their products taste better and promote additional consumption.[24]

In short, the body wants what it wants, and it does not have a magical mechanism for obesity prevention. Neither do dogs, by the way—animals that are suffering their own obesity crisis and will eat chocolate with abandon even though it is toxic for them. Canine bodies have no more wisdom to prevent obesity than human bodies do. Obesity rates prove that our tastes are pretty basic, and in this land of constant plenty, most of us are going to gain weight.

There is no magic mechanism, but there is consciousness. Later in this chapter we will provide advice on how to think your way past your baser food desires.

The Highly Palatable Painkiller

To reinforce just how profound the effect of highly palatable food is on the pleasure centers of the brain, it's worth pointing out that such foods can actually dull or at least distract us from painful experiences. Doctors use the tactic of placing a little sugar solution into a newborn baby's mouth before taking blood to prevent or at least mollify the patient's wails.[25]

The hormonal alchemy of sucrose placed on the baby's tongue activates a dopamine rush in concert with an opioid effect that masks the sense of pain associated with the needle.

Let's drive home with some imagery that point about intuitive eating being a crock. We're born to love sweetness and have to learn to appreciate bitterness (like what is found in vegetables).

To prove it's innate, Margaret put her scientist cap on and she experimented on her friend's baby (with parental permission, naturally) while I snapped photos.

"Sugar elicits a feeling of pleasure," Margaret said. "We tell that by the baby's smiling."

This is the happy face of the five-month-old baby girl after having a sugar solution placed on her tongue:

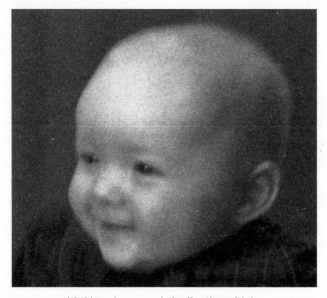

It's blurry because she's vibrating with joy.

"Bitter tastes," Margaret said, "unfortunately send a message to the brain that you're eating something poisonous, so the reaction is crying and fussing. Historically, vegetables were not worth our time to eat because they lacked energy density, which is why the learning process to accept vegetables is difficult."

And so, this is your kid on spinach:

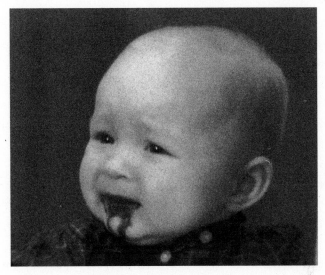

Why are you doing this to me?

Mixing Uppers and Downers into Tasty Speedballs

In case we haven't made it clear: obesity is caused to a significant degree by pleasure-focused eating. This is the "hedonically motivated" kind of consumption where we lose control because the food tastes so good, making those reward pathways in the brain commence firing away like a scatter gun at a hillbilly BBQ.

Pleasure is the result of a kind of chemical alchemy traced to two major hormones in the brain: dopamine and opioids.[26] Dopamine and opioids are involved in the sensation and expectation of pleasure, and we experience a surge in both when we eat junk food.

A "speedball," in drug vernacular, is a mixture of an "upper," in the form of cocaine, and a "downer," in the form of heroin or a like substance.

The Upper: Dopamine

It can be hard to unlearn what you have learned.

Last week, my wife went to Costco and bought a giant tin of Almond Roca for stocking stuffers.

Uh, hello? IT'S MONTHS UNTIL CHRISTMAS! This is like buying Halloween candy in August.

I know there is Almond Roca in my house. ALMOND ROCA IN THE HOUSE! I know where it is. I know it's on a shelf down in the basement right next to the dryer. I know the container is pink and cylindrical and has a gold plastic lid. I can see the shape and size of the golden-foil-covered treats inside. I could draw one from memory. I know what it's going to taste like. I know it's there. I know it tastes good. I know I want it. The pleasure centers in my brain have burned all of this into memory.

Excuse me for a moment.

Oh, wow. That was good. And now, a message for my lovely wife: WHAT THE HELL WERE YOU THINKING? Do you believe there will be ANY of those left by the time Christmas arrives?

I do love her, so I won't blame her. I'll blame dopamine (and opioids) instead.

The role of dopamine has been the focus of scientific debate, and while it is still under investigation we know it plays a part in pleasure, learning and craving. When a survival-enhancing behavior is completed, dopamine is fired. Engaging in rewarding behavior increases the level of dopamine transmission in the brain and this directs our attention toward things that make us feel great.[27]

Dopamine also fosters a strong positive memory; it encourages our search for rewards that elicit the most pleasurable experiences.[28] That's why I know so much about Almond Roca, and why I can draw an accurate map from memory of every fast food restaurant within a five-mile radius of my house, and yet I can only guess at what vegetables are in my fridge right now.

Dopamine is what makes us crave highly palatable food. Its firing goes beyond the sensation of pleasure experienced when eating that food to include the *encoding into memory* of that experience so we will seek out such foods again in the future.

One of the reasons it's difficult to control these cravings is the expectation of the reward we'll receive once we satisfy them. We *know* food X, Y or Z is going to taste good, so we want it.

The Downer: Opioids

Opioids are another kind of neurotransmitter that helps determine food preference. The weight of scientific evidence on the subject supports opioids enhancing the pleasure factor of eating, making the experience more rewarding and causing people to seek out such effects again and again *despite* the known negative consequences associated with doing so (such as weight gain).[29]

Opioids are responsible for the hedonic impact of food.[30] Just as the heroin (an opiate) in a speedball produces euphoria, so do things like chocolate. But as Leigh Gibson pointed out in chapter 1, the euphoric effects of junk food are short-lived.

And these buggering opioids are even more nefarious. They act within the brain's reward pathways in ways that *inhibit* satiety.[31] This means that foods high in hedonic value—the ones that taste best—trigger a response from opioids that not only say, "This is awesome," but also insist, "No, we're not even close to being full. Keep shoveling more in."

Chocolate: The Socially Acceptable Speedball

"I hate chocolate," said no one, ever.

Chocolate is one of the most craved substances in the United States.[33] The inclusion of caffeine in the mixture accounts for some of this, but the draw is mostly due to the mixture of sugar and fat. Each on its own is rewarding enough, but merge them into one treat and it's a recipe for neurochemical reward pathways run amok.

Eating a sugar-fat combination, like chocolate, activates both dopamine and opioid circuits in concert. You have the upper and the downer effect at the same time. Although the effect is not to the same degree, chocolate is like a legal, socially acceptable speedball. Sugar is the cocaine giving you the "high," and fat is the heroin giving you that relaxing, euphoric "mmmm."

It's a compelling sensation, and it makes you want more. The opioids say what you're doing is pleasurable and therefore must enhance survival, and the dopamine says the body is getting what it needs—energy—so that must enhance survival too.[34]

"The most powerful foods are the ones that combine sweetness and fat," Leigh Gibson told me. "We do find with stress eating that chocolate is the number-one preferred food."

You probably knew that already.

It's worth noting that the discovery of the opioid systems stems from the use of opium. Go figure. Morphine is the most active ingredient of opium and remains a popular painkiller despite an array of adverse side effects (drowsiness, tolerance, dependence). Heroin was synthesized from morphine and today is a main illicit drug of abuse.

ADHD and the Risk of Obesity

ADHD—attention deficit hyperactivity disorder—can make you fat. Look! A puppy!

"There are strong links between ADHD and obesity," Carolyn Davis told me. "Those who are more inattentive are more impulsive." And impulsivity translates to a higher ingestion of palatable food. "Another reason is the lack of planning associated with the disorder and the need for immediate gratification."

Harvard neurologist Dr. Miguel Alonso-Alonso agrees. "We know that people with ADHD have higher rates of obesity than the rest of the population," he said. "Impulsive people have more acute responses that are more driven by the environment." And the environment is rich in highly palatable food.

Medication can help, but so can exercise as a tool to ameliorate impulsivity.

Opiates stimulate the opioid system; highly palatable food stimulates the opioid system.[32] Got it? Scary, right?

HIJACKING THE REWARD SYSTEM

So now you know that just because something feels good doesn't mean it's good for you. Scientists refer to behaviors or substances that elicit extreme reward—by releasing an unnatural amount of dopamine and opioids on ingestion—as being capable of hijacking the reward system.[35]

The natural foods consumed by our ancestors didn't pose this problem. The opium poppy doesn't mess with you the way its refined street version does. Even the marijuana of yesteryear pales in potency compared with modern-day ganja.

Humans messed with food and drugs and made them all way more powerful, and that added power is now screwing with our brains. Recall the question I posed earlier: how many calories of mangos can you eat in one sitting compared with calories of carrot cake à la mode?

The Dopamine Tsunami—Too Much of a Good Thing

Scientists believe that, just as happens with certain drugs, consuming too much highly palatable food will dim the dopamine receptors.[36] The dimming or pruning of dopamine receptors leads to an enhanced tolerance for junk food, which leads to wanting more junk food. The end result? A situation in which you only feel like eating junk food and end up gaining weight as a consequence.

How does this happen? Imagine an ocean. Now imagine a forest right next to this ocean. When you ingest substances (such as foods high in sugar and fat) that release a massive "wave" of dopamine, this wave acts like a tsunami. It crashes into the forest (where the trees are your dopamine receptors) and wipes out a bunch of trees.

But we need those trees. They're an integral part of the overall eco-system known as your brain and body. If there are enough dopamine tsunamis, more and more of the trees/receptors get knocked down. They're overwhelmed and destroyed, leaving behind a barren landscape.

And it gets worse. Now that your body and brain are used to these massive, havoc-wreaking surges of dopamine, it takes even more of the original substance to create the same-sized tsunami, and there are fewer and fewer trees left to absorb it. This is what you call a vicious circle.

Ever hear of drug abusers first taking the substance to feel good but then building up a tolerance to the point that they need more and more of the drug to achieve the same effect? After a while, the poor souls are taking the drug just to *stop* feeling bad. The same thing can happen with food.

Here is what the vicious circle of food compulsion looks like:

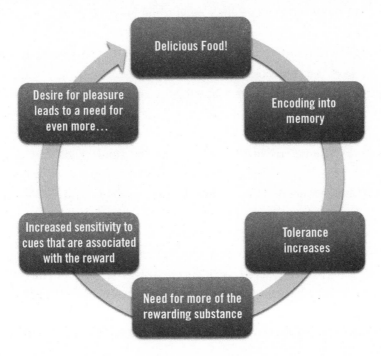

"The more you overeat energy-dense foods," Eric Stice says, "the less reward you get and the more you need to eat to get that reward. You need a larger and larger dose."

This phenomenon is called raising the reward threshold. Cocaine does it. Heroin does it. And building research suggests that too much highly palatable food does it as well.[37]

A 2001 study published in the *Lancet* showed brain scans of 10 obese men and women and 10 controls. It found that dopamine receptors were decreased in obese individuals in direct relation to body mass index. The authors compared frequent consumption of highly palatable food to alcohol, cocaine and opiate abuse and found the effect on dopamine receptors to be similar.[38]

And a 2012 study of 151 healthy-weight adolescents published in the *American Journal of Clinical Nutrition* found that frequent consumption of ice cream, independent of body-fat levels, resulted in a reduction in "reward-region responsivity in humans, paralleling the tolerance observed in drug addiction."[39]

· In other words, you don't need to be overweight before the dopamine receptor pruning begins.

"The system that suppresses impulses to overeat is a limited resource," Dr. Alonso-Alonso told me. "These areas of the brain can be exhausted quickly. We are overusing the control systems because of the current environment."

Dr. David Katz, founding director of the Yale University Prevention Research Center and an authority on nutrition and weight management, sums it up nicely: "The food industry, when they said, 'Bet you can't eat just one,' weren't kidding around."

Do you now see why you need every tool you can muster, such as integrating exercise into the equation to help you control food cravings? (We'll cover how exercise affects appetite in chapter 4.) I'm good at managing food intake, as is evidenced by my four-pack abs (hey, if I was great at it I'd have a six-pack), and yet I have a hard time resisting that Almond Roca stash because I know I have 24/7 access to it. If it weren't in the house, the desire to go get some would be manageable. Successful resistance involves removing temptation. In a 2013 study published in *Neuron*, Molly Crocket, a neuroscientist at University College London, and her colleagues describe this as "precommitment," which is a "voluntary restriction of access to temptations." The research team found that such precommitment is a far superior dietary strategy than willpower in the face of temptation.[40]

When someone is kicking the heroin habit, you don't put her or him in a house full of heroin. This is why a key component of getting off junk food is avoiding it as much as possible. When you stimulate the opioid system in addition to eliciting dopaminergic activity—a consequence of eating junk food—we've got to do better than just out of sight; the junk's got to be so far out of reach that seeking it out represents enough of a pain in the butt to cause you to rethink your desire.

Why There's Always Room for Dessert

One of the best meals I ever had was on a cruise ship. It was all just so good and I stuffed myself to the gills. I couldn't eat another bite.

And then the crème brûlée showed up.

I ate it.

This is sensory-specific satiety in action. It refers, in scientific terms, to the declining satisfaction generated by a specific type of food the more you eat of it, and the consequent appeal of a new food that allows you to keep eating once full of something else.[41]

In a 1986 article in *Nutrition Review* on the subject of sensory-specific satiety, Professor Barbara Rolls reports that "the pleasantness of the sensory properties of the eaten food decreases significantly more than the pleasantness of uneaten foods." Rolls explains that this effect is greatest when the uneaten food is different in taste type to the eaten kind. In other words, a sweet dessert is always an option—even after a big steak.

This biological process is also advantageous from an evolutionary standpoint. "Sensory-specific satiety helps to ensure the consumption of a varied, and therefore balanced, diet. Thus, when a variety of foods are available, there will be a tendency to switch from one food to another because of the decrease in palatability in any one food after consumption," reports Rolls.[42]

A number of other studies show that the more variety you have in your food, the more your satiety signals will get overridden and allow you to keep consuming past fullness.[43]

In a land of overwhelming choice and abundance, it's all those options that encourage you to overeat. The stereotypical buffet feeding frenzy is just one example of the ways in which we override the system and consume far more calories than are needed to maintain body weight.[44] Limiting your access to this endless variety is one strategy for controlling consumption. Another is retraining your brain, on several levels.

Doing It Doggie-Style

Sorry, bad analogy. When I was a kid I saw my standard poodle eat until he puked, then eat the puke.

Pavlov's dog: ring a bell and he salivates. Why? Because Fido had been conditioned to associate the bell with food.

Weaning yourself off junk food is all about retraining your brain, and that requires breaking with your past conditioning. We learn to like certain foods through this conditioning: we taste something, it's rewarding (yummy!), and we remember it.[45] *Jersey Shore* notwithstanding, we are the most advanced species on the planet thanks to the complex nature of our brains. We have an immense capability to remember associations between a certain food and the time, place and conditions under which it was consumed.[46]

When I smell candles being blown out, I think birthday cake. Hell, when I use the big Black & Decker massager on my neck and, after a while, it makes the same ozone smell as the mixer in my kitchen, I think birthday cake.

The principle of food reward gets exploited by pervasive advertising: grocery stores, TV, radio, online, magazines, newspapers . . . it's everywhere. Images and advertisements about food send a powerful message to the most primitive parts of the brain, the same parts that are geared toward survival and don't, therefore, take into account whether we *need* to eat.[47] For most of human history we gorged when we could to put on lifesaving fat stores for a future famine. It didn't matter if we weren't hungry. The people who were best at this survived. And we descended from those survivors. Unfortunately, food advertisers take advantage of this survival mechanism.

Dairy Queen, Alice Cooper and the Fire Woman

My wife was out with the kids one day and I was watching TV; a Dairy Queen commercial for the Blizzard came on. I'm not much for Blizzards, but an image of the Peanut Buster Parfait entered my brain (that recall, by the way, was dopamine in action).

My kids are allergic to peanuts. On the rare occasions when we do take them to DQ I can't have the one thing I long for, but the two trouser trophies weren't around this time . . .

I was up and out the door in seconds; it wasn't until I hit the drive-through that I realized I'd left my wallet at home. Not to be undone, I remembered the change drawer in my car (more dopamine at work, enhancing working memory to obtain the reward)[48] and scrounged enough to pay for the tasty treat.

After annoying the teenager at the drive-through window with a handful of quarters, I parked with my Peanut Buster Parfait and commenced inhalation. *Nights with Alice Cooper* was on the radio; he played "Fire Woman" by the Cult. The song lasted longer than the dessert.

That day, I fell victim to a food cue—the damn TV commercial—that had an immediate effect, prompting me to go buy a specific product. But cues go *way* beyond that in how they affect eating behavior.

YOUR BRAIN ON FOOD CUES

Cues aren't just about the visual, like seeing the McDonald's Golden Arches or watching a TV commercial. There are also a variety of sound cues—from corporate jingles to sizzling bacon[49]—and olfactory cues can be overwhelming[50] (but I find those Cinnabons never taste as good as they smell). Cueing can even be situational; if you eat in front of the

TV or in your car, engaging in television watching and driving can create an unconscious cue to consume food.[51]

We're eating all the time, and part of the reason is that we're *reminded* to eat all the time.[52] Food is big business, and that industry's advertising budget is second only to the automotive industry's. We have billboards, television, radio, magazines and newspapers, the Internet and mobile apps, sights and sounds and smells and a culture that is all about food, food and more food. Seriously, the next time you're watching TV, pay attention to just how many of the commercials are for food.

"We've experienced that showing children food commercials stimulates eating behavior," said Emma Boyland, an experimental psychology researcher at the University of Liverpool. "It also shifts their preferences toward types of food shown in the commercials." It works on the category level, where McDonald's commercials elicit higher fast food consumption. "Everybody responds to advertising," she said. And yet kids don't even know that they're being persuaded.

Out of Sight, but Not Out of Mind

Those prone to overeating have a tendency to ignore the future consequences of doing so, such as weight gain. And studies have shown that people who have less self-control are more vulnerable to temptation when it comes to highly palatable food.[53] Interestingly, these temptations don't have to be in the form of actual food. The treats do not need to be readily available when the craving begins.[54]

And we don't become immune to these cues, either. "After repeated exposure to cues we don't develop a resistance to them," Boyland said. "Instead, we become more sensitive to them."

And so we eat.

What Exactly *Is* a Food Cue?

A cue is not food; it is a *representation* of food.[55]

"Food cues are about associative learning," Eric Stice told me. "The more you pair Hershey's Kisses with their tinfoil wrappers, the more tinfoil by itself will make you think of chocolate." And it can be as subtle as a color. Think of the shade of purple that Cadbury uses for its Dairy Milk chocolate bars. Seeing a woman wearing a dress of that same shade can make you crave chocolate, and you don't even know it's happening.

It can even be a letter, like an *M* making you think of M&M candies, or, if someone wrote the letter in a way that looked like the Golden Arches symbol, of Big Macs. Toddlers can learn to recognize the letter *M* long before they learn their ABCs simply because they've been to McDonald's enough times.[56] That's bad.

More often than not, however, cues are pictures of delicious food.[57] DQ sundaes on a billboard. Skittles falling from the sky in a commercial. Steaming French fries in a magazine ad. Fresh doughnuts in a website image. I've posted photos of my barbecuing prowess on Twitter and Facebook. Last night I wanted to show how puffy my Yorkshire puddings were, and that went on Facebook too. I didn't even stop to think about how I might be part of the problem.

Even restaurants are using images with increasing frequency. Margaret told me of a recent experience while dining out: the server brought an iPad to the table to show off pictures of the various desserts they had available. Items oozing chocolate, glistening with caramel, sprinkled with bits of toffee . . . Just writing about it makes me want them.

The point is that if you're thinking about food, you're going to want food. And we live in an environment where you're forced to think about food.

The Effect of Cues on Appetite

The more sensitive you are to the rewarding effects of food, the more motivated you'll be to seek it out,[58] and the more motivated you are to seek it out, the more likely you are to eat it. And the more you follow through on these cravings, the more the pattern is reinforced.[59]

The issue with food cues is that over time you begin to pair the food reward with the signals and symbols (the cues) that express its location and availability.[60]

Remember all that dopamine stuff? It's a key ingredient in this phenomenon.

For our Stone Age ancestors, dopamine encoding of memory was valuable for remembering which pools and streams had the most fish, where to find the most nuts and berries and the migrating patterns of prey. But how is dopamine involved with seeing a *picture* of food?

It all links back to the effect on memory. When we see an image of tasty food, we are reminded of its rewarding effects, and this builds a greater sense of anticipation and desire for that feel-good sensation. Dopamine enhances this sense of anticipation further. Researchers call the effect the *theory of incentive salience*, which explains how those who are the most likely to crave food are also the most vulnerable to developing patterns of overeating.[61]

"It's Pavlovian conditioning," Carolyn Davis told me. "When Pavlov paired food with the bell, the dog learned to salivate just when the bell was rung even though no food was present." Our cue-rich environment means the bell is always ringing, and it prompts us to action.

"The more you eat palatable food, the more your brain becomes hypervigilant to seek it out," Stice told me. "If you regularly eat fried food, the *smell* of fried food will initiate a higher craving much more than in someone who doesn't consume such foods."

Incentive salience suggests that our motivation to obtain a reward is distinct from our sense of pleasure associated with that reward.[62] Some people are more vulnerable to the rewarding effects of drugs not because they *like* them more but rather because they *want* them more.[63] This makes sense: while pretty much everyone likes chocolate, some people *crave* it.

Motivation Run Amok

A Dairy Queen commercial made me get in my car and drive three miles for a dessert. The cue motivated me to go. As we've noted, dopamine also played a role by making sure I knew not only where the DQ was located but also the fastest route to drive there.

The more people crave something, the more motivated they are to obtain it. It's no longer simply a matter of food being present and engaging in opportunistic feeding (like the buffet); the cue itself prompts action. Plenty of us will go out on a chocolate or ice cream run to satisfy a craving. Often these cravings are the result of a cue, and the target doesn't even realize that he or she has been manipulated. He thinks it's just a random craving that popped up, but it wasn't random at all.[64]

Interestingly, though, cues can have the opposite effect to the one intended. During the 1980s, Nancy Reagan, the US president's wife, launched a popular "Just say no to drugs" campaign that used images of drug paraphernalia as part of its attempt to show the dangers of drug use. The problem was that the needles and crack pipes featured in advertisements and on billboards elicited a craving for drugs among users; incentive salience meant that such ads contributed to *more* drug-taking behavior, not less.[65]

And what can we say about a diet program or book that shows piles of sugary and high-fat foods—meaning to present them as something negative or something to be avoided? Not surprisingly, such images can actually *increase* the longing for those food items. The book *Wheat Belly*, by cardiologist William Davis (a book we do *not* recommend; you'll learn why in chapter 5), has a stack of bagels on the cover. Davis unfairly demonizes wheat while simultaneously failing to understand that by having a pile of wheat products on the cover of his book he's creating a longing for it in his readers every time they see the image.

BREAKING THE ASSOCIATION: TRAINING YOUR BRAIN

We'll spend a lot of time in Stages II and III sharing ways in which you can counteract the conditioning that's gotten you into this mess in the first place. Our Virtuous Cycle diet and fitness plan breaks it down step by step.

For now, understand that an important part of limiting your junk food intake will involve reducing exposure to the prompts that make you crave it. If you're not being reminded of junk food, you'll consume less of it. Logical, yes, but is it always practical? After all, you do have to live in this obesigenic world, where food cues are abundant. That's why we'll also work on strategies and skills for how to deal when you *can't* avoid the prompts. Exercise is a big part of this. You'll see why in chapter 4.

In the meantime, here's one important bit of information: if you're well fed, you're less sensitive to food cues,[66] which is why you should make sure you've eaten before going to the grocery store. It makes that trip through the checkout line with all the chocolate bars and potato chips more tolerable. (Conversely, people who are hungry or have been on a restrictive diet for a prolonged period are more sensitive to cues.)[67] One trick I use to avoid even *looking* at those treats is to read the headlines on gossip magazines instead; it allows me to feel superior.

But it goes beyond hungry versus full. Some people are more sensitive to cues. A 2012 study published in the journal *Obesity* used fMRI technology on 49 individuals and showed differences in brain reactions to food imagery between lean and obese subjects. The latter revealed much higher activation in the reward-sensitive areas of the brain when shown images of junk food. Interestingly, when images of bland foods were shown, there was no difference in the brain activation between lean and obese subjects.[68]

And this is the part about this study that is going to blow you away. Pay close attention to what this means, because it's damn important.

Those 49 people were in three groups: obese, normal weight and successful weight loss maintainers (SWL). The fMRI images of the SWLs showed greater activation in the frontal regions of the brain, which are responsible for future planning and decision making, when shown images of highly palatable food. This part of the brain is also responsible for "inhibitory control," which means it's a source of willpower when it comes to not acting on impulses, like the impulse to eat junk.

What this means is that these successful weight loss maintainers were using *higher brain functions* to think their way past the cue and not let it prompt them to desire food. They had *trained their brains* to defend against eating junk food.

And here is the killer point, which is a teaser for chapter 4: exercise strengthens the hell out of this region of the brain and its ability to function in this manner. *The hell*, I say!

If you begin to lose weight via dieting alone, the power of cues *increases*.[69] We just mentioned that people who are hungry or dieting are more susceptible to the power of cues. Well, guess what? When you lose weight via a restricted diet *combined with exercise*, the effect of cues either remains the same or diminishes.[70] This is why chapter 4 is going to be like a giant, gooshy Valentine's Day love letter to exercise.

YOUR BRAIN ON ALCOHOL

Before moving on to the bigger picture of a healthy lifestyle, let's wrap up the brain science with a final topic.

Oh, and . . . *hypocrisy alert!*

I drink. Sometimes I drink too much. I've bailed out on more than one workout due to a hangover.

Okay. Now that that's out of the way . . .

The Alleged Benefits of Alcohol Consumption

Moderate alcohol intake might be good for you, but studies extolling its virtues for preventing heart disease do not qualify as concrete proof. The studies are not controlled and randomized but instead rely on self-reporting of alcohol intake. What's more, they often lump ex-drinkers (who are often people who have had a drinking problem in the past and can have a host of other bad habits) and lifetime non-drinkers into the same "abstainer" category.[71]

According to a 2005 study in *Sports Medicine*, "Available evidence suggests . . . moderate alcohol consumption may have favourable effects on blood coagulation and fibrinolysis [whatever that is—I think it's good]; however, compelling experimental evidence is lacking to endorse this."[72]

In short, when it comes to the question of whether alcohol can be good for your heart, the answer is, we're 100 percent certain that we're just not sure. However, we know for sure that what *is* good for your heart is exercise. Speaking of which . . .

The Effect of Alcohol on Exercise

When it comes to exercise, booze is not your friend. Have you ever tried exercising with a hangover? It's no fun.

But it's worse than that. According to the same 2005 study mentioned above, alcohol decreases athletic performance because it "adversely

The Calories! Oh, the Calories!

Booze has calories, lots and lots of calories:

Description	Serving Size	Approximate Number of Calories
Red or white wine	5 oz	120
Most beer	12 oz	150
Most spirits (no mix)	1 oz	65
Most liqueurs	1 oz	100

Alcohol calories rival that of sugar-sweetened beverages, which make up approximately 6 percent of Americans' daily energy intake. A 2012 study of 11,000 US adults by the Centers for Disease Control and Prevention found that alcohol calories account for roughly 5 percent of total energy intake.[74] Liquid calories are not satiating, and high ingestion is a major cause of weight gain.

affects energy supply and impairs the metabolic processes during exercise." Chronic use also causes muscle fiber wasting, and that's bad too.[73]

Temporary Euphoria, Bad Calories

Earlier in this chapter, we explained how highly palatable foods give you a brief boost of euphoria; the mood-boosting effects of alcohol are more significant and do last longer, but the crash is harder too. A bad hangover is about as euphoric as a barf-coated shovel to the head.

It gets worse.

According to a 2001 study in the *American Journal of Clinical Nutrition*, "increasing alcohol consumption was associated with a higher total energy intake."[75] That means more calories, but not just any calories—bad calories: more animal products and saturated fat and fewer vegetables.

"After a few beer the ability to make wise food decisions goes down," said Richard Mattes, a professor of nutrition science at Purdue University. A number of other studies support the idea that alcohol has an appetite-stimulating effect, and can therefore lead to weight gain.[76]

So if you drink, you take in a bunch of alcohol calories and you've also got that "decreased inhibitions" thing going on. That same alcohol-infused behavior that causes you to French your co-worker at the office Christmas party is also what makes you think deep-fried cheese sticks will really hit the spot.

Okay, I know you're going to have a difficult time accepting this, but I interviewed Jenni "JWoww" Farley of *Jersey Shore* fame (or is that infamy?) on the subject of how drinking can lead to grease inhalation.

"For season one of *Jersey Shore* all the partying led to lots of late-night snacking," she told me. "Because of the alcohol I'd be eating pizza, Philly cheese steaks and cheese balls. Oh, God, I love cheese balls." Tell me about it. "There were also days of being too hungover to go to the gym. After the first two seasons I hit a wall. I couldn't fit into my pants anymore and I decided to clean up my diet a little and become more health-conscious."

Cheesy cheese ball cliché alert! If JWoww can realize the booze is making her eat bad things and resolve to change, so can you. If you like the stuff, keep it moderate. Check out the sidebar to the right for some tips on how.

Tips for Taking It Easy on the Ethanol

- Do you really need to go to that party/bar/get-together? Only go to parties you actually want to attend.
- How about volunteering to be the designated driver now and again? You still get to go to the party and have fun, but you know ahead of time that indulging isn't an option.
- Club soda is your friend; it looks just like a gin and tonic. No one will know.
- Make your drink last. Don't chug.
- Delay drinking. Don't reach for alcohol early in the evening; wait until the party or event is in full swing.
- Drink water in between alcoholic drinks. You'll imbibe less and be less dehydrated, which means a reduced hangover.
- If you're entertaining, ask people to take leftover booze home with them or find alternatives to give it away.

SKILL POWER MORE THAN WILLPOWER

Man, so much doom and gloom. You're probably right freaked out by it all. Perhaps you're thinking, *How can I possibly find the will to resist this world of constant, overwhelming food and drink temptation?* The answer is that resistance is more about building skills to navigate the modern food environment than relying on sheer determination and grit.

"Skill power is like riding a bike," Dr. David Katz said. "At first it's intimidating, but once you know how to ride it you wonder what all the fuss was about." I'll note that Katz is one of the sanest people I've spoken to on the subject of weight loss.

But what about willpower?

"There is far too great an emphasis on willpower." Willpower is still an important component, Dr. Katz affirmed, but it's not the be-all and end-all. "Everyone who wants to lose weight has the will to do so. Do today's seven-year-olds have less willpower than the ones from 50 years ago? The obesity epidemic isn't a result of a loss of willpower," he said.

It's pairing willpower with the necessary skills that makes exercise and healthy eating sustainable. "These things can happen by a force of will, but it's difficult to sustain," Katz said. Conversely, "When you have a skill, you have it forever."

Katz asserts the need for a "tool kit" for healthy living. He is also an accomplished carpenter. He explained that in order to build something, he needs both the appropriate tools from his shop *and the skills to know how to use them.* Otherwise, that jigsaw could result in some missing fingers.

Make no mistake: there are tools needed to lose weight—things such as guides to deciphering food labels and counting calories, as well as exercise equipment and workout clothes. But these need to be coupled with the knowledge of how to use them, not to mention a firm grasp on planning and time management. These, too, are important skills that make sustainable weight loss possible.

"Skill power paves the way," Dr. Katz said.

When it comes to highly palatable food and its cues, it can seem as though your brain is your enemy, making you eat at an unconscious level, and that's true. The trick is to become more conscious and use your higher cognitive capabilities to think your way through this—to use those "skill powers" that Dr. Katz describes to reduce the effect of cues.

This book is all about making you skilled at managing your weight. As you now should know, it goes far beyond the rudimentary mathematics of eat less, move more. These are skills for living, and you can master them. In Stages II and III, we'll show you how.

We're smarter than dogs. Just because the bell rings doesn't mean we have to salivate.

3

WHY YOU SHOULD BE
EXCITED TO CHANGE

We cannot change anything unless we accept it.
Condemnation does not liberate; it oppresses.

—CARL JUNG

Passion is superior to fear as a motivation to change. That's why this chapter will focus on the positive outcomes you can achieve from exercise and healthy eating. Nevertheless, we still need to cover some of that doom and gloom stuff about being sedentary, eating junk and having excess body fat. It will help you understand why it's so important to make the effort.

THE GOOD NEWS
Insert random motivational "you can do it" statement here.

Seriously, once you get into the groove of healthy living you'll discover numerous reasons beyond looking and feeling better that keep you going, such as . . .

Adding to Your Life Résumé
If you're overweight and don't like being so, that's a problem—one that's difficult to solve. But if you do it—if you work hard and persevere and achieve your goals—you will have gained tremendous experience as a problem solver. And that's a skill that can be applied to myriad aspects of your life.

There's even proof. Albert Bandura, an internationally renowned behavioral psychologist and Stanford University professor, examined this phenomenon with the development of his groundbreaking self-efficacy theory. According to Bandura's theory, sustained weight loss is a "performance accomplishment." And repeated success (or accomplishment) makes it easier to deal with occasional failures. And overcoming these failures "can strengthen self-motivated persistence if one finds through experience that even the most difficult obstacles can be mastered by sustained effort."[1]

Am I the only one who said, "Hell, yeah!" after reading that?

Those performance accomplishments build on one another. If your life could stand some improvement, getting in shape does *way* more than give you a healthier and hotter body to live inside. It gives you the mental discipline and willpower to kick more ass at the rest of life. It's your return on investment.

It gets better.

Fitness ROI

Even though pursuing fitness costs money, time, effort, sweat, pain and smelly laundry, it can pay you back financially. Yes, *financially*. And I'm not just talking about the qualitative stuff like improved health, longevity, physical performance, appearance and self-esteem. There are hard numbers to run here, such as what happens when you compare people who exercise at least three times a week with those who exercise less (or not at all).

"I found that for men the average was a 6 percent increase on weekly earnings. For women it was more on the order of a 9 to 10 percent increase in weekly earnings." Vasilios Kosteas, an associate professor of economics at Cleveland State University, told me this.

Kosteas's study, published in the *Journal of Labor Research* in 2012, controlled for things such as education, age, gender, health status and body weight to make the exercise probability as close as possible.[2]

"These results support that there is a causal relationship for exercise increasing income," he said.

But why?

"We have a good body of evidence that shows exercise is linked to having greater energy levels, better cognitive function, improved mood—all of these things lead to greater performance at work, and greater confidence as well."

So there you go. By taking some time away from your career to focus on health, you can actually enhance your career. Who knew? But before we talk about how great your life can be, we need to talk about . . .

Taking Shame Out of the Equation

You're probably familiar with a whole range of "yo mama so fat" jokes, but how many have you heard about how black, gay or Jewish "yo mama" is? Why is making fun of the overweight still okay?

"There is no question that the stigma and bias and discrimination surrounding obesity is the fairest game," says Dr. Yoni Freedhoff. "In popular culture the vilification of obesity is constant, whether it's obese characters who are lazy, clumsy and gluttonous, or the types of responses to public policy statements about dealing with obesity."

Freedhoff told me that these responses stem from a simple fact: most people erroneously believe that the overweight are somehow choosing to do this to themselves. They think if we'd just push away from the table we'd all be slim.

What a crock.

In 2011, the International Diabetes Federation released a position statement to combat the common belief that obesity is the result of a personal failing or lack of motivation, writing that "this perspective ignores the very strong genetic and developmental bases to severe obesity compounded by physical, emotional and societal issues."[3] The statement also explained that obesity stigma leads to discrimination at work, socially and even in the health care system.

This is not the way to motivate people. In fact, a 2012 study by researchers in the Department of Psychological and Brain Science at the University of California, Santa Barbara, found that people who experience stigma over their weight experience elevated stress, which reduces self-control, which in turn can lead to weight gain.[4] In a 2013 paper published in *PLoS ONE*, researchers from Florida State University were more damning, asserting that not only does stigmatizing obesity lead to poorer mental health outcomes, but the authors stated that "rather than motivating individuals to lose weight, weight discrimination increases risk for obesity."[5]

Again, when obesity is stigmatized, *it causes weight gain.*

Kris Beneteau, 48, is an office worker in Windsor, Ontario. At her heaviest she weighed 271 pounds and had to face a lot of stigma both for being overweight and for choosing bariatric surgery (which we'll cover in appendix B) as a tool to combat her condition. Now maintaining at 145 pounds, she told me how poorly people treated her when she was heavier.

"There was definitely a stigma attached," she said. "Once, a stranger told me I shouldn't be in a Baskin Robbins to get ice cream, like it was somehow his business."

And no matter how talented or accomplished a person may be, for some, only that extra weight is visible. In 2009, Brent Smith, lead singer for the multi-platinum-selling band Shinedown, was on *The Today Show*. Right before his performance, host Kathie Lee Gifford said, "At first I thought he was Meat Loaf," and her co-host Hoda Kotb laughed aloud at the gibe. I asked Brent how that made him feel.

"It really stung," Smith told me. "I'm a fan of Meat Loaf, but she wasn't talking about a musical comparison. It was national television and my heart kinda fell on the ground . . . It was like the performance didn't even matter. It was a tough comparison for me that morning."

The jokes aren't so funny for those who are the brunt of them.

Fat shaming leads to extreme dieting, depression, eating disorders and more. Wendy Williams told me her parents called her fat all the time when she was growing up, and it led to decades of disordered eating.

Don't listen to the shamers. You can't adopt exercise and change your eating behaviors if you have a toxic mind-set. Hating your body is not a healthy way to approach changing it. If you don't exercise, I'm not going to blame you for not being active, and you shouldn't blame yourself. This is *not* about blame but about ownership. You are the 100 percent undisputed owner of your body, and if it's in poor shape, no one suffers more than you. Your body is where you live; it's home sweet home until the day you become worm food.

So give yourself a hug, because it's time for a bit of doom and gloom before we get to the good stuff.

THE BAD NEWS

Being sedentary, having a poor diet, smoking and being at higher-stage obesity are all leading causes of early death. This last item is a *major* risk factor for all forms of heart disease, stroke, type 2 diabetes, certain forms of cancer and a host of other debilitating conditions such as mental deterioration, gout, gall bladder disease and sleep and mood disorders.[6]

The longer you stay glued to a couch, the greater the risk of death from myriad causes, agrees Bill Kohl, a professor of epidemiology and kinesiology at the University of Texas at Austin. And the older you get, the more infirm you become. "Continued inactivity into the 60s and 70s results in balance insufficiencies and lack of strength," Kohl told me. "Daily living becomes much harder."

Science Trumps Circumstances

Prior to the 20th century, lifestyles were much different than they are today, as most labor was done by human power rather than machines. People didn't need jogging shoes or gym memberships; they busted their butts all day long just to make a living. Diets were lower calorie and not full of refined, high-calorie food, and few people were overweight. Back then we ate for fuel to live; today we eat mostly for pleasure.

And still, the poor buggers dropped like flies. Average life expectancy prior to the 20th century was less than 40 years of age.[7]

Don't start celebrating. Yes, we live longer lives now, but this is *in spite* of our terrible lifestyles. We have modern medicine, adequate nutrition and clean water to thank for improved longevity. Rates of death from heart disease are declining, even as obesity rates, sedentary living and overconsumption of unhealthy food rises, but this is because of improved medical treatments.[8] But now a major health care crisis is looming. In the not too distant future the whole medical system could become overwhelmed if people don't start focusing on preventative medicine rather than treatment.[9]

BMI—Bogus, Maligning Information?

Margaret and I struggled over whether to even include BMI—body mass index—in this book. Yes, knowledge is power, but this knowledge probably doesn't really help you, because it attaches labels like "obesity"—not a nice-sounding word—to people. Labels are not always a true measure of health, and they certainly don't represent individual differences in lifestyle or amount of muscle. Higher levels of body fat are but one piece of a large and complex puzzle.

There's ample evidence to show a person who is physically active on a regular basis and eats a quality diet can still be "overweight" or even "obese" and live a long life.[10]

"Exercise trumps a lot of other bad behaviors," Dr. Michael Joyner, a physician-researcher and expert in exercise physiology at the Mayo Clinic in Minnesota, told me. "Large people who are very physically active are only at a slightly increased risk of all-cause mortality and cardiovascular disease compared with those who are lean and fit." But those who are large and sedentary are at a two to four times risk, he says.

But still, excess fat creates cause for concern. There are those who say it's no big deal, but let's look at the evidence.

A 2013 meta-analysis published in the *Journal of the American Medical Association* showed that while more severe obesity was associated with higher mortality, being overweight or in a lower stage of obesity was actually associated with a *lower* overall mortality than a "healthy" body weight.[11]

The media went nuts over this study, yet there's a mighty "but" that goes along with that analysis. Problem number one is that the study looked only at death rate and not illness. We may be living longer, but we're not living better. Medical advances can keep us alive even while we're carrying around unhealthy levels of body fat, but there is a significant difference between joyous living and mere existence.

Excess body fat is often inversely proportional to vitality. There is merit in questing for its reduction.

Problem number two is that the study didn't adjust for the fact that people often lose a lot of weight when near death. It also didn't correct for alcoholics, drug users or people with eating disorders, all of which can inhibit weight gain. In other words, the study didn't compare these overweight and mildly obese people with those in the normal weight range because of a healthy lifestyle. It's not a realistic comparison.

So what happens when there is a realistic comparison? What happens when you control for things such as smoking and history of disease? Well, a 1999 study in the *New England Journal of Medicine* of *a million people* did find that the risk of disease and death from all causes increases as weight goes up.[12]

What's more, a 2013 study published in the *American Journal of Medicine* asserts that "the dangers of obesity have been grossly underestimated in clinical outcome studies because of the failure to control for cigarette smoking, inappropriate control for the biologic effects of obesity (e.g., hypertension and diabetes), and failure to exclude subjects at baseline with severe weight loss due to subclinical disease."[13] The author notes that obesity was approaching smoking as the leading cause of avoidable death worldwide.

Fit and Fat

Even so, excess body fat by itself does not spell disaster. As Dr. Joyner said, exercise is a good trump card. I asked my wife, a family physician, what she's thinking when she sees an overweight patient. "If the person is overweight but doesn't smoke, exercises, has good blood pressure and cholesterol levels, I don't worry about it too much," she told me. How you live your life has far more impact on your health than the number on any scale.

Unfortunately, most people—overweight or not—do not follow healthy lifestyles. In fact, only 23 percent of Americans engage in the barest physical activity to garner *minimal* health benefits.[14] Additionally, in 2010 the Centers for Disease Control and Prevention estimated that only 24 percent of American adults consume the recommended five or more servings of fruits and vegetables a day.[15]

Blood Type: Gravy

And know that just because someone looks fit doesn't mean the person is healthy.

Do you remember that 1970s TV classic *The Partridge Family*? Former child star Danny Bonaduce grew up to have a stint on reality TV with *Breaking Bonaduce*, and viewers often saw him shirtless and revealing a muscular and chiseled physique. He was also a heart attack waiting to happen.

"The doctor said my blood was 'like sludge,' and I told everyone my blood type was 'gravy,'" Bonaduce said to me. "My cholesterol was 357, like the Magnum."

A total cholesterol level of 357 (9.23 for my fellow Canadians) can be just as deadly as a pistol. Bonaduce earned his number by drinking to excess, smoking and taking anabolic steroids. Someone with much higher body fat but with healthier habits would have a longer life expectancy.

THE *WHY* OF HEALTHY LIVING

Enough of that. Sorry for bumming you out. The good news is this: if you take gradual steps to transform your body into a lean and powerful machine, you get to live in a nicer metaphorical house. Actually, forget the house analogy; houses don't move.

Let's talk cars instead.

Imagine someone who never exercises. She's in bad shape. She has no energy. She's overweight. In the automotive world, her body is a rusted-out old Pinto towing a rickety U-Haul. Now imagine what she feels like when she trades that car in for a brand new Porsche (no U-Haul). Can't imagine what it feels like? Well, I can tell you it's friggin' awesome.

You may be old, morbidly obese, injured, sick and screwed in the genetic lottery, but you can still ditch the clunky old Pinto. You may never get a brand new Porsche, but most people can achieve a low-mileage Honda. Maybe even a slightly used Lexus.

Trading Up

So how do you get yourself into that Honda or Lexus? As I mentioned at the beginning of this chapter, fear isn't going to help you. It can motivate people for a short period of time, but it has no staying power. The key to long-term success isn't fear—it's passion. So use the doom-and-gloom information as a small part of that initial thrust to get yourself moving, then focus on moving ahead rather than looking back. Don't think about what you're doing as giving up something bad; think about chasing something good. There is good news in all this.

"It's never too late to start exercising," Kohl said. Interestingly, these are the exact words the original fitness guru, Jack LaLanne, often repeated before his death in 2011—at age 96. "We've learned that even the oldest of the old can increase their muscle mass. Even at 90," Kohl said.

"There are few things that physical activity doesn't help in terms of health," reports Kohl. "It is remarkable for preventing falls and therefore risks of broken hips." The functional health benefits from becoming a regular exerciser are tremendous for aging populations.

Speaking of Jack, I interviewed his widow, Elaine, who told me of his endless enthusiasm for helping motivate people to move. "He wanted to show people that just because you're older it doesn't mean that you have to give up," she said.

Five years from now you could be feeling 10 years younger. I could compose a mighty tome about the benefits of healthy eating and exercise alone. There is a pile of research big enough to choke an interstellar sandworm. When I write "studies show the benefits of healthy eating and exercise," I'm talking about something on the order of forty-eleven gajillion studies, and we've listed a micro-percentage of these in the next endnote about how exercise and healthy eating, as well as abstinence

These Boots Are Made for Knocking

Let's talk about sex, baby.

Ooh, Salt'N'Pepa flashback.

"Exercise is good for overall sexual performance," says Emily Morse, a sex expert, Bravo TV personality and author based in San Francisco. "If you're strong and in good shape you're going to be able to perform better," she told me. "More important, lack of self-esteem is a big killer of sex drive, and it's often tied to body image issues."

"The most basic part is that when you feel better about your body, how it looks, feels and works for you, you're just going to have better sex," agreed Maryanne Fisher, a professor of psychology at St. Mary's University in Halifax and a specialist in sexuality research. "You're going to be less self-conscious and more able to be connected to your partner."

Beyond the psychology, there's also physiology.

"The better shape you're in the more you can sustain the activity," Fisher told me. "You can have a longer sexual encounter. We know that someone who exercises gets libido-boosting effects and fewer erectile problems."

Research supports this. If you either own a penis or enjoy using such equipment, know that being obese and in poor physical condition increases the risk of erectile dysfunction between 30 and 90 percent.[17] Lean and fit men aren't the ones who need Viagra.

from smoking and avoiding excessive alcohol intake, dramatically improve quality of life and longevity.[16]

Wouldn't you like to be stronger, able to run faster, have better endurance and more energy? Following the advice in this book will get you there. How about getting sick less often, sleeping better and being happier about your physical appearance? This book leads to that too.

And speaking of being happier, your brain and mood get a boost, and stress decreases too (we'll cover that in chapter 4).

Compressed Morbidity? That Doesn't Sound Good

Actually, it *is* good.

We've got mega endnote 16 about the increased longevity that comes from living healthily, but guess what else happens? You go downhill fast! *Hooray!*

Seriously, hooray! This is *good* news. Think about it: Say you get yourself into awesome shape and live to 90. Wouldn't you rather be spry right up to 89? The whole "falling apart just to let you know death is looming, so make your peace" messaging takes maybe a year, and then you're fertilizer. Cue Elton John: "It's the circle of liiiifffffeeee . . . and it rules us aaaaalllll . . ."

Okay, maybe that sounds less than awesome. After all, we're talking about the Big D here, and it's coming for you. It's coming for us all.

Man, I suck at this. Back on track. You want to know how most people die these days? Not that rainbows-and-puppy-hugs version I showed you up there, that's for sure. They're dying way younger than those who live healthy lifestyles, and after an extensive downhill slide to boot. They suffer longer. By comparison, people who take good care of themselves not only live longer, but they get a lot more life, quite literally, out of their years. The nosedive into dirt nap is mercifully brief.[18]

Biology > Machinery

Yeah, I'm going back to the car thing, but only to tell you why humans are more awesome than BMWs.

Your body is the opposite of a mechanical machine. When machines are pushed to their limits and used for long periods day after day, they wear out much faster. In animal biology, however, the opposite happens. Machines don't have the capability of self-repair built in. We do.

When we challenge our body with physical activity, we send it a message that says, "I expect more." The body answers by adapting to the new challenge. Systems are activated right down to the cellular level to make you better.

Unfortunately, it works in reverse too. When you sit around, you break down.

No matter how bad your level of fitness is right now, you can improve it. Maybe one day science will discover the fountain of youth in a pill, but that is a *long* way off. For now, there is only one fountain of youth, and we'll show you how to find it in Stage III.

You need to be thinking long term. Humans are programmed for instant gratification, but planning for the distant future can make the difference in your golden years between climbing Mount Kilimanjaro and puttering around a retirement home on a motorized scooter.

I said death is coming for us all, but that doesn't mean you can't fight it.

Blood and Creative Juices Flowing Together

I am Best. Dad. Ever.

The day I interviewed singer Sarah McLachlan also happened to be my daughter's 12th birthday. Did I mention that my daughter worships Sarah? After the interview McLachlan got on the phone with my little girl and wished her a happy birthday.

Now, go clean your room.

No one would question McLachlan's creativity, and a 2012 article published in *PLoS ONE* determined that being physically active out in a natural environment boosts creativity because it is an "emotionally positive" experience, but also "low arousal" when compared with things such as television and Internet, which inhibit creativity.[19] I know about half of this book was written in my head while in the saddle of a bike, and I mentioned this research to Sarah to see if she had similar experiences.

"I totally agree," McLachlan told me. "Running is very rhythmic and I have written a lot of lyrics while out running. It's a very musical exercise, and sometimes I like to sing when I run. Your whole body is doing the same thing. I'd much rather be in the expanse of the wilderness because it feels like part of my world. It's a unique perspective. You're this tiny speck in a huge environment and it's nice to be reminded of that."

McLachlan also likes surfing, but I expect that, in the interest of safety, her mind is more focused on the task at hand while riding waves.

The Valiant Delaying Action against Age

Train hard enough and you'll peak eventually. I haven't hit my peak yet. I've still got that Ironman on the bucket list. Hopefully a Boston Marathon qualification too.

We all get older. The tough ones don't let it slow them down. Neil Peart is not slowing down.

Peart is the drummer for the legendary Canadian rock 'n' roll group Rush. In 2011, *Rolling Stone* named him the greatest drummer alive. "Playing a three-hour Rush show is like running a marathon while solving equations," he told me right before the band's penultimate performance of its "Time Machine" tour in Vancouver. "My mind is as busy as it can be, and so is my body—full output all the time."

Peart is dedicated to maintaining his endurance. He's fighting a valiant delaying-action against age.

"I have to pretty much not ever get out of shape," he said. "The stamina aspect is great because you don't lose that with age so quickly. I know there will be a day when I just can't do it, but at 58 years of age it hasn't come yet. I can still play as fast and as powerful and as long as I ever could."

My best friend and I watched him perform his drumming marathon from the front row that night. Neil was telling the truth.

A FINAL WORD OF ENCOURAGEMENT

You could be facing a turning point in your life.

Let's leave science behind for a moment, and I'll just give you some good old-fashioned advice.

Maybe your life is a crud sandwich. Alternatively, it may be excellent and the only part missing is a healthy body. More likely is that you fall somewhere between the two. Things are okay, but they could be better.

You may feel there are things you should be doing with your life. You may have a list of unrealized ambitions, half of which you've forgotten. There is a nagging itch in the back of your mind that you're supposed to be doing something more, something *better*. So here's my real-life advice: *don't give up on this.*

Persevere at getting in shape, because it is going to make everything else in your life better. At the very least, it will make things suck less. Don't discount that, because sucking less is often the first step in getting better.

Remember what I wrote earlier in this chapter about physically active people making higher salaries on average? It's because they have the added energy, confidence and a positive outlook on life that promotes ambition. Such people chase their dreams and are more likely to achieve them.

Getting in shape changed my life for the better in ways beyond measure. I wasn't in a full-on death spiral when I took the plunge; I just wanted to ask my girlfriend to marry me. She was light-years out of my league, and I wished to minimize the chances of her saying no when I handed her a sparkly little rock and asked her to please put up with me forevermore.

I knew she wasn't shallow like that. I just wanted to look good and be healthy for her. Considering a proposal of marriage seemed like a good impetus to change. And so I did.

There are a number of things Fit James ended up doing with his life (so far) that I'm certain Unfit James never would have accomplished.

Oops. Apologies for the Bob Dole moment, but perhaps if I stick with third person the following will seem informative and not conceited.

Fit James completed two master's degrees and had a successful business career. Fit James worked his butt off to become a syndicated columnist for the *Chicago Tribune* and *Los Angeles Times*. Fit James's soul mate said yes to the sparkly rock.

Living a healthy lifestyle isn't easy, but it has a benefits package that is second to none. As you'll see in the next chapter, it's not just your body that changes for the better but your brain, and that's pretty awesome.

It's not an instantaneous change, though. All these positive outcomes emerge at what may seem like a snail's pace, which is why patience is key.

I'll say it again: don't give up on this. Slow progress is still progress.

4

WHY YOU *MUST* EXERCISE

A strong body makes the mind strong.

—THOMAS JEFFERSON

John Lennon was right: all you need is love—the love of exercise.

Exercise is a key tool for fighting food cravings and changing eating behaviors. When it comes to weight loss, burning calories is helpful, but it is a *distant second* to the psychological, hormonal and chemical changes that exercise initiates—changes that allow you to gain control over what you eat. Getting physically active is *the most powerful* tool there is for controlling eating behavior.

Are you an inactive couch potato? Do you hate the idea of sweating? I understand, because I used to be the same way. I was the high school spaz who made the geeks look good and always got picked last when teams were chosen. I sucked at every sport imaginable, yet I now love exercising almost every day of the week. I have about 50 pounds less fat and 20 pounds more muscle than I did two decades ago.

This isn't "if I can do it, so can you" motivational pablum. I hate that. I just want you to know I have some perspective on what you're about to go through.

EXERCISE IS CRITICAL

"Exercise is a critical component of weight loss and weight mainte-nance," Dr. Miguel Alonso-Alonso, who specializes in how exercise affects the brain, told me. "We know that. It's a fact."

Harvard doctor up there. He says it's critical. Take heed.

I'll be blunt. You'd be a fool to ignore exercise as part of your weight loss strategy, because it creates a suit of armor to protect you from the endless temptations of our toxic food environment.

Why am I harping on this? It's because I've been to the bookstore. By my estimation, 80 percent of weight loss books are either only about diet or pay the barest lip service to physical activity. They perpetuate a myth that exercise is torture and sweating is gross. Well, sweating *is* kind of gross, but you get used to it, and there are breathable fitness clothes that mitigate its ickyness.

Miracle-diet books that promise "no exercise required" are telling people what they want to hear. Instead, I'm going to tell you what you *need* to hear. (What this will mean for book sales remains to be seen.)

Exercise improves diet, which reinforces exercising, which improves diet, which . . . creates a *virtuous* cycle. When it comes to health and fit-ness, would you rather be in a virtuous cycle or a death spiral?

A word of caution before you dash off to the gym or the pool or the cross-country skiing trail: while exercise is indeed rewarding, the most important thing to remember when adopting an exercise regimen is to avoid the trap of the reward mentality. We're talking about the state of mind that leads some people to burn 300 calories on a treadmill, feel they've earned a reward and then eat 500 calories' worth of cheesecake. That's bad math.

Understand that exercise is not about allowing you to reward yourself with junk food but about giving you the power to RESIST junk. You need to embrace the lifestyle rather than see it simply as a means to an end.

EXERCISE AND COGNITIVE CAPABILITY

Actor Jesse Eisenberg's character in the movie *Zombieland* extolled the virtues of "cardio" as an apocalyptic survival tool. I'll bet it never crossed his mind that all that activity was making him a more scrumptious target for the walking dead.

All supposing a better-functioning brain is also a tastier one, that is.

Decreasing Deterioration

I love *The Simpsons* and always laugh when Grandpa has a "senior moment." But it's not so funny to imagine it's you getting senile. A little later in this chapter, we'll get into how exercise pumps up your cognitive capabilities (and how this affects food intake), but first let's examine how both resistance training (like weightlifting) and aerobic exercise can ward off a host of neurological impairments.

"It's a medium-sized effect—but since we're talking about the brain, medium is good," Michelle Voss, assistant professor of psychology at the University of Iowa and lead author on a 2011 review of the effect of exercise on cognition, told me.

I'd say very good.

Exercise as Therapy

Margaret and I are not experts in how to deal with a traumatic past or stressful situations, but we do know one thing: food is not the answer. Neither are drugs or alcohol.

We have bad days, bad bosses, bad childhoods and thus bad cravings for eating junk. But it's important that you don't use the latter to medicate any of the former. The best healthy escape from a life that feels as if it's sucking you dry is exercise, though a healthy sex life can help too.

If you've got some serious I-feel-messed-up-in-the-head issues, you may want to seek professional help and deal with these problems at their core. We wish you success and happiness; know that the information in this book can be used in conjunction with your therapy.

However, if you don't believe psychological intervention is required, we offer an alternative: exercise therapy. It worked for me and it works for Margaret.

It's worked for millions; people have created a positive relationship with exercise to give them something to feel good about. You too can wash the pain and stress away in a pool of sweat.

Voss and her team examined more than one hundred studies on the topic and discovered interesting things. Here's one: the brain benefits of resistance training seem to differ from those you get from aerobic exercise.[1] "Aerobic exercise improves ability to coordinate multiple things, long-term planning and your ability to stay on task for extended periods," she said. Resistance training, which had been studied much less than the aerobic side of things, "improves your ability to focus amid distracters."

This makes sense to me: aerobic exercise such as running involves staying on task for a long time, and if you're training to get better, you need to stick to a plan. Weightlifting requires ignoring the spandex and lousy gym music and focusing enough to prevent the barbell from crushing your trachea during bench press.

The details of what's going on inside your skull are fascinating. Voss explained that the fMRIs of people in their 60s showed increases in gray and white matter after just six months of exercise. This increase happens in the prefrontal lobes (which control decision making) and temporal lobes (which control sensory input), sites that typically diminish with age. With exercise, Voss told me, they grow.

Voss also explained that the hippocampus area of the brain, key for memory formation, shrinks 1 to 2 percent per year in those older than 60. But when people in this age group begin fitness regimens, it *grows* by 1 to 2 percent instead.

Beyond growing one's brain, exercise improves the ability of different parts of the brain to work together, Voss says. It talks to itself better, but not in a multiple-personality kind of way.

Exactly how hard were the researchers pushing these over-60s? I could see how the excitement over the results might be curtailed if one had to become a power-lifting marathoner to reap benefits. But that's not the case. Simple brisk walking for 45 minutes three times a week gets results.

And, Voss added, going much beyond that won't give your brain much more: "There definitely is a law of diminishing returns. The difference between zero and moderate exercise is significant, whereas the difference between moderate and high exercise is much less so."

Exercise also can help if you've got a genetically programmed Alzheimer's time bomb ticking away in your noggin. In 2000, Dutch researchers published a study of 347 men, some of whom were genetically prone to Alzheimer's due to a certain gene variant. Adjusting for a number of confounding factors such as smoking, drinking and education, the researchers found the inactive couch potatoes with the brain-wasting gene variant were *four times* more likely to develop Alzheimer's than the fit people who carried the trait.[2]

Genetic tendencies aside, exercise reduces your risk of developing silent brain infarcts. And if you surmise that a "silent brain infarct" is something unpleasant, you're right. It's also called a "silent stroke." It's a lesion. On your brain. That's bad.

In 2011, Columbia University researchers published a study of 1,238 elderly people in the journal *Neurology*, reporting that the 25 percent who were the most physically active were nearly half as likely to suffer these brain lesions compared with their inactive counterparts.[3]

Cerebellums and cerebrums and medullas, oh my!

As we learned back in chapter 3, scare tactics are lousy motivators for just about anything, including diet and physical activity, so let's just forget all that doom and gloom stuff. (If you have the Alzheimer's gene variant, forgetting should be easier . . . I know. I'm going to hell.) Since fear isn't going to get your butt in gear, let's get deeper into the benefits of how exercise both reduces stress and enhances brain function in myriad ways.

Chilling Out with Cardio

Do you ever feel like making a voodoo doll in the image of your boss, stabbing it full of pins, twisting its head off, then setting it on fire?

I remember those days.

Speaking of the old days, here's to the good old mammoth-slaying Stone Age, when we really knew how to deal with stress. I'm talking about the fight-or-flight response, an inherited advantage coded into our genes via natural selection. Say you were chillin' at the cave one day when in sauntered one of those saber-toothed murder beasts. The resulting stress would have elicited a massive surge of adrenal hormones; you'd jump to your feet and go all caveman on the intruder with valiant stabbing or cowardly fleeing.

Either way, the hormone surge was short-lived. Soon enough, you'd be roasting up tiger steaks or muttering about how you didn't like that cave anyway as you headed off in search of a new abode to drag Daryl Hannah back to.

Fast-forward a few millennia, and it's goodbye murder beast and hello performance reviews conducted by supervisors with double-digit

IQs. And as good as it might be for stress relief, you can't kidney-punch a domineering boss, throw him out a high-rise window and declare yourself alpha drone o'er the cube farm. Hooray for progress.

Instead, you send a snotty email to some unsuspecting IT guy about how your stupid keyboard isn't Diet Coke–resistant, or yell at a slow driver from the safety of your minivan during the commute home. And when you finally get back home, you pour yourself a stiff drink and crab at the kids to stop doing those things that kids do before you collapse in front of the TV to watch your favorite team lose or see *The Bachelor* give the boot to the one woman you thought deserved to win his heart.

Also, you eat. Remember all that stuff in chapter 1 about stress-induced eating? Stress does not lead to healthy food choices.

But it doesn't have to be this way. Casually flipping through a 2006 copy of the *Annals of the New York Academy of Sciences*, I learned that exercise is the key to combating the stress of modern life.

The authors, from the University of Ioannina in Greece, first explain (in regard to the fight-or-flight response) that "stress responses can be elicited by emotional stimuli or professional and social stress." No kidding. Just one negative memo handed down from on high can get the glucocorticoids and catecholamines flowing, but since you just sit there and stew, these adrenal hormones go unused. Your body stores them in visceral fat deposits, and this does bad things to you.[4]

The article then describes how these stored adrenal hormones disturb gonadal function (no wonder Viagra is such a big seller) as well as growth hormone and thyroid function. The authors explain how these "metabolic disturbances" lead to "comorbidities including central obesity, hypertension, dyslipidemia, and endothelial dysfunction."[5] In other words, unrelieved stress turns you into an artery-clogged hippopotamus with Limbaugh-like blood pressure and a lousy immune system. Oh, and it's also hard on your brain.

The aforementioned cavemen didn't have to worry about heart disease and senility. They became food for something else long before their arteries clogged up or their brains turned to tapioca. For real, this time: hooray for progress!

Continuing on in PhD-speak, the authors inform us that "accumulating evidence documents the beneficial effects of regular exercise in preventing or ameliorating the . . . comorbidities induced by chronic stress."[6]

There's that word "comorbidities" again—you want to avoid those.

The American Psychological Association has also weighed in on the subject of exercise and stress, noting online that "physically active people have lower rates of anxiety and depression than sedentary people." This mood boost probably has nothing to do with that old myth about exercise unleashing a surge of happy-making endorphins, the statement adds, since there's not much evidence for this popular belief.

Still, the effect may be more than just chemical. "Exercise seems to give the body a chance to practice dealing with stress," according to the APA. "It forces the body's physiological systems—all of which are involved in the stress response—to communicate much more closely than usual."[7]

We can sum up all this science talk as follows: not only is stress killing you, it's making you fat, which is also killing you. You can't beat up your boss, but you can whale on a squash ball or pound the heck out of a pair of running shoes.

So try that instead, and stay employed.

Sweating Out the Sad

Maybe stress isn't your big issue. Maybe you're seriously bummed out instead, perhaps even clinically depressed. If so, you should know that a host of recent research affirms the antidepressive effect of exercise.[8] Depression overwhelms people. Even a mild case taxes your neurological capabilities, making wise food choices all the more challenging.

"We find the remission rate of depression in the highest exercise dose was right on par with the use of SSRIs [antidepressant medication]," Dr. Tim Church, an expert in exercise and health at the Pennington Biomedical Research Center, told me. "This was about 200 minutes per week at a moderate intensity."

What Church's research is telling us is that just over three hours of exercise a week at moderate intensity is an equivalent treatment to antidepressant medication. This doesn't mean we should all flush our doctor-prescribed pills, but it does say a thing or two about the ability of physical activity to improve your mood.

Actor Mariel Hemingway says exercise saved her life.

"I suffered depression most of my life, and fitness and eating well have been very important in terms of battling this," Hemingway told me. "My mother had cancer and my dad had heart disease and people were fighting all the time and there was a lot of alcohol. And being out and moving in nature is what made me feel complete and whole." It's worth noting that Mariel has lost seven family members to suicide. "[Exercise has] been very important in helping me get through those darker times," she said.

"Exercise has a lot of benefit to the brain," Dr. Church said. "With neural imaging looking at before and after exercise, we're seeing changes in volume and size of the brain. It seems like reducing insulin has a positive effect on the brain." Church explained that a molecule associated with improved brain health and repair is increased by exercise, and this molecule is also associated with lower levels of stress, anxiety and depression.

"People report exercise as being a good way to cope with stress," Leigh Gibson told me. And he expands on Church's comments on insulin: "There is literature developing that links insulin resistance [which can lead to type 2 diabetes] to poor appetite regulation." Professor Gibson explained that because exercise is powerful for controlling insulin sensitivity, it's an additional mechanism for controlling what you eat.

"It can definitely regulate mood," the professor and obesity researcher Carolyn Davis says of exercise. "It can make you feel better, more energized, and can help you concentrate so you don't need the distraction of nibbling on something."

Pumping Up the Cognitive Capabilities

In 2011, researchers from the University of South Carolina put 35 subjects on treadmills in order to figure out what exercise does for building mitochondria in the brain. If you remember middle-school biology, you'll recall that mitochondria are the powerhouses of the cell because they provide most of its supply of chemical energy.

Granted, these "subjects" were mice, and that's just as well, because the researchers then dissected the rodents' brain tissue and examined the differences between treadmill-aficionado mice and cage-potato mice. Lo and behold, eight weeks of treadmill running made mouse brains more fatigue-resistant due to an increase in mitochondria.[9] The little quadrupeds had pumped up their cognitive capabilities.

In Search of Happiness

Tomes abound on how to find it, but for many, happiness eludes. I believe it arrives via an indirect route. Physical activity elicits a physiological response that decreases stress, improves mood and battles depressive feelings. And from a psychological perspective, it's hard not to smile when you've modeled your physique into something healthier that performs better, something you're proud of. Make yourself proud.

Michelle Voss explained that increased mitochondria improves the brain's ability to get blood and oxygen where it needs to go. "There is a shorter refractory period as well." Translation: you recover more quickly; periods of mental exhaustion are shortened.

This comes in handy. When I go for a long run, cycle or other workout session, it's my brain that pushes me. I have to resist my legs, which are saying (or shouting), "Dude, we're done." My brain drives them by replying, "No, keep going." When your body is screaming at you to stop, it takes an effort of will to override that. I believe this mental aspect of exercise is primary in continuing to push yourself even though you're tired.

And yes, this mental toughness comes in handy for sticking to a healthy diet.

HOW EXERCISE AFFECTS EATING BEHAVIOR

It's time for this chapter to get climactic.

So far we've explained that exercise prevents brain rot, chills you out, creates feelings of happiness and makes your brain fatigue-resistant. All this contributes to you becoming a better eater, yes. There is less stress to promote emotion-based eating, and you have the mental energy to choose your foods wisely.

Hang on, it's about to get even more awesome.

"Physical activity and eating behavior are connected in the brain at the cognitive level," Dr. Alonso-Alonso told me. "They share the same mental processes."

I promised awesome, but awesome requires a bit of explanation, so bear with me.

Alonso-Alonso explained that we use goal-oriented systems in our brains to suppress impulses to eat junk food. Remember in chapter 2, when we talked about how higher impulsivity leads to higher body weight? In order to lose weight, we need to suppress that impulsivity. "The resources for goal-oriented eating behavior are greatly enhanced via physical activity," he said. "Exercise improves eating behavior through brain and cognitive changes."

Exercise enhances the brain's "executive function," which is what allows you to follow a plan. Sticking to a healthy diet means sticking to a plan. It's about adherence to goals. You have to resist urges too, but mostly it's about following a healthy eating plan.

So what is executive function? Dr. Alonso-Alonso explained that it's located in the prefrontal cortex and is a combination of three things: your ability to control impulsive behavior (like the impulsive desire to reach for that doughnut), adaptability and working memory. These three things working in concert form your decision-making capabilities.

"There is a dose-response effect," Alonso said. "A fitter person is going to have greater improvements in executive function and therefore better control of what they eat."

Every time you eat, you're making a decision, or decisions. Salad or hamburger? Takeout or home cooked? Not surprisingly, higher executive function = better decisions. Oh, and according to Brian Wansink, a professor of consumer behavior and nutritional sciences at Cornell University, *we make over 200 decisions about food every day*.[10]

Giving Senior Management a Support Team

Executive function is the senior management of your brain—and the folks in the corner office of your cerebral cortex have a tough job.

Alonso-Alonso co-authored a 2011 paper in *Obesity Reviews* explaining that the modern environment—not just from a food perspective but from an *everything* perspective—tires out our executive controls on a daily basis.[11] These controls are of a limited capacity, and the obesigenic environment means they are taxed. Eventually, the repeated need to control impulses becomes too much and we give in.

And by give in, I mean pig out.

That poor senior exec is overworked and, honestly, starting to suck at his job. He needs help. Enter exercise. Exercise is like giving the guy a *venti* Starbucks brewed by a barista who switched the caffeine dial to "weapons grade." Except, unlike with coffee, you don't get the crash. Or the spaziness. As mentioned earlier, being physically active chills you out. What I meant with the whole java analogy is that your poor, suffering decision-making capabilities get a significant boost from exercise. It's like hiring a highly qualified assistant to keep that executive on task. Higher awareness and goal-oriented thinking is key to sticking to a diet. There really is a think-yourself-thin component to weight loss. But there is more to exercise than pumping up the cognitive capabilities. It also works on . . .

The Unconscious Level

Exercise makes you jones less. I wish the Joneses in my neighborhood would teach their stupid dog to shut up.

I digress. By less jones-ing I mean less craving, and not just food craving. Got a thing for the ganja and trying to cut back on your Visine usage? In 2011 researchers from Vanderbilt University in Nashville put a dozen potheads on treadmills and made them run for 30 minutes 10 times over a two-week period (I can just imagine the barfing-up of lung tissue that resulted). These were heavy users, and they saw a dramatic drop in both their cravings and their usage (a decrease of more than 50 percent) after just a few exercise sessions.[12] Exercise was the *only* intervention. What's especially interesting is that these people were deemed cannabis dependent, and didn't even want treatment to help them stop smoking pot. But the exercise alone made them cut their marijuana use by more than half. Okay, maybe the coughing-up of alveoli while on the treadmill played a role, but note that the cravings were reduced as well.

And this goes way beyond the stinky green stuff. A 2011 analysis of the research published in *Frontiers in Psychiatry* revealed that exercise is a powerful tool for reducing self-administered use of a host of other mind-altering substances, including cocaine, meth, nicotine and alcohol.[13]

And this is why exercise is used in treatment for addictions.

"Patients work out with us every day," Jennifer Dewey, fitness director for the Betty Ford Center in Rancho Mirage, California, told me. "It's a mandatory part of the treatment program." Betty Ford offers a wide variety of exercise opportunities, from outdoor activities such as hiking, biking, kayaking and rock climbing, to personal trainers and a yoga studio.

"It's one of the critical components of sustaining sobriety," Dewey said. And it's not just while in treatment. "We give them routines they can take home and follow." They help patients plan for a fitness-focused future as an aid to stay clean.

How does physical activity help people break bad habits? It's because exercise is a replacement reward. It's hitting the same neurochemical pathways in the brain as things such as booze, drugs and even gambling. Back in chapter 3, we met Shinedown lead singer Brent Smith. He used exercise as his replacement reward to kick the booze habit. Coupled with cleaning up his diet, this led to tremendous weight loss for the rocker.

"Exercise can release opioids in the brain and be reinforcing," Nicole Avena told me. "It's hard for people to get to the point where it's reinforcing, but after a while they crave it." Yep. No one likes running the first several times they do it, but you've got to power through. Pretty soon you'll look forward to your run in the same way you used to look forward to a bag of Doritos.

Speaking of which . . . exercise has the ability to reduce cravings for junk food as well.[14]

Working Up a (Loss of) Appetite

Have you ever heard the expression "work up an appetite"? Yeah, that doesn't actually happen. There are people out there who will tell you that the effort you put into exercise is wiped out by an enhanced appetite, therefore making physical activity useless for weight loss. Don't listen to them; it's just another form of snake oil. They're telling you what you want to hear: *Weight loss can come with no effort required. Buy my product.*

Story time again.

Through an amazing case of serendipity, I had a mandatory work event at the same time as my wife's cousin's wedding on the other side of the country. She took the kids, and I had a few days of bachelorhood. I also had some nice weather, and one day I pushed myself further than I ever had on my bike, riding it for six hours solid. That evening was meant to be a gluttonous feast of beer, pizza and high-definition violence on my big-ass TV as loud as I damn well pleased.

Um. Not quite. I could barely stomach two beers, and I didn't order the pizza. I made a salad and

Help for the Reward Sensitive

Some people are reward sensitive. They are more likely to be addicted to food, alcohol, drugs and even gambling. I spoke with actor Daniel Baldwin, who has been on both *Celebrity Rehab* for his drug and alcohol addiction and *Celebrity Fit Club* for being obese.

"I'd just turned 50, weighed 285, and my doctor had read me the riot act about my health," Baldwin told me. He started intense training with a kettlebell, which led to dietary improvements, which led to losing 50 pounds in six months.

"My doctor didn't recognize me," he said. "He thought I was Billy Baldwin."

Daniel says he loves working out with kettlebells because it's fun and allowed him to lose fat and build muscle. He also says the confidence boost that comes with his new physique has been good for battling his addiction demons.

"What this does for me emotionally, psychologically and spiritually . . . has been very important in not relapsing," he told me.

In other words, Daniel started getting his fix from working out. You can too.

a salmon sandwich and could not finish them. I was just not hungry or craving beer, even though it was a rare night without husbandly or parental duties—plus I was getting to watch movies of bullets ripping through soft tissue, swords cleaving body parts and stuff getting blowed up. It was family-guy nirvana.

But that intense effort of a day on the bike resulted in an anorectic effect. This is not to be confused with anorexia, which is bad. What it means is that all that activity suppressed my appetite. I have noticed this effect many times after aerobic activity such as running, cycling and swimming, and it can last for much of the day. My six-hour ride is an extreme example; it doesn't take nearly that much effort for the ano-rectic effect of exercise to kick in. A big pile of research supports the appetite-suppressing aspects of moderate physical activity.[15]

Interestingly, it seems to be mostly aerobic exercise that suppresses appetite, and not resistance training like weightlifting.[16] As someone who is avid for both activities, I can attest to the veracity of this research. Uh, I mean, yeah. That seems about right. Research also shows that the more intense the exercise, the more profound the appetite-suppressing effect.[17] That also seems right.

"Exercise is good to control appetite," Avena said. "It releases hor-mones that are associated with satiety. You have a reduced desire to eat."

Oh, and sitting around all day doing nothing doesn't cause you to eat less.[18] So much for that theory of "working up an appetite." It's ironic that burning extra calories has the power to make you ingest fewer calo-ries, but there it is.

Regrowing the Dopamine Receptor Forest

Cast your mind back to chapter 2 for a moment and recall all the dopa-mine tsunami doom and gloom. The dopamine receptors are a forest that gets washed away with wave after wave of highly palatable tsuna-mis. And pretty soon you're craving more and more of whatever your "highly palatable substance" is to get the same effect.

Evidence shows that exercise helps those receptors grow back.

A 1994 study published in *Brain Research Bulletin* determined that both synthesis and metabolism of dopamine have a close relationship with exercise. It makes these receptors more effective.[19]

And more recently, we have rats on meth. A 2012 study in *Synapse* let rats go on a meth bender, which must have been hilarious to watch, and it burned out their dopamine and serotonin receptors. After getting their chemical freak on, some of the rats were left to be cage potatoes, and others were made to run. The results show that the running rats significantly reduced the meth-induced brain damage, and that all the activity had a profound positive effect on their dopamine and serotonin receptors. And the lazy rats? Well, let's just say it sucked to be them. The Swiss-cheesing brain effects of the dope lingered.[20] Truthfully, it sucked for both groups. They all got their brains dissected.

Exercise can lead to a greater concentration of dopamine receptors (which are more sensitive). This, in turn, is tied to a reduced need for overconsumption of highly palatable food—your sensitivity to reward is higher, so it takes less of whatever it is you're ingesting to make you feel good. When it comes to reward-seeking behavior, a little bit of junk food will go a long way.

Sweet, Sweaty Memories

All the positive benefits of exercise that we've discussed so far have been physiological, but there is also an important psychological link between exercise and what you eat.

What I mean is, if you begin making a big effort with exercise, do you want to undo it all by eating a bunch of crap? The answer for some people is yes, I earned it (we'll deal with that at the end of this chapter). For many, however, exercise is the beginning of a subtle change in their relationship to food.

"When you exercise, it creates a life perspective where you don't want to undo it all with an unhealthy diet," Eric Stice, the eating behaviorist, told me.

Knowing that you exercised makes you think more about consuming healthy foods that will feed your recovery. Knowing that you're about to exercise makes you yearn for foods that improve performance. Seriously, I like doughnuts, but if I'm about to work out, a Boston cream is the last thing I want. And forget about *during* exercise. In the middle of my workout, a doughnut or other fatty, sugary treat could make me blow chunks. In my experience, an exercising stomach is finicky about what you put in it before a workout.

And there are studies that show exercise works as a gateway behavior (something that leads to adoption of a new behavior)—on the psychological level—for healthier eating.[21] On an anecdotal level, the majority of the people I spoke to for this book about their weight loss journeys attested that it was exercise that transformed the way they thought about food. Cheryl Berube is one example.

A 43-year-old graphic designer in Nova Scotia, Berube has had issues with emotional eating ever since she was a child. "I used to hate running and now I really love it," she said. "I was always overweight as a child and never thought I would ever run." But she did, and it changed her eating. "I think it reinforces better eating. I noticed when I do my normal exercises I don't tend to snack in the evening, which is my worst problem." The result? A whopping 160 pounds lost via simple diet and exercise, and she's keeping it off.

Remember Jen McKinnon? She told me, "All this exercise has put me in the right mind-set for dealing with food. When my kids were driving me nuts, I'd go for a run instead of going for the chocolate."

"I fell into a big slump after university and I was eating crap all the time," Jessica Banas, a 24-year-old office worker in Ontario, told me. "I gained about 40 pounds." And, to toot my own horn, Jessica told me she read one of my articles about viewing food as fuel for exercise and started walking. Her knees didn't like that, so she switched to cycling. "It was love almost right away," she said. "It became my thing. I definitely consider what I eat before I cycle now. Being a dedicated cyclist means being careful about my diet."

When it comes to eating, Dr. David Katz refers to exercise as "the wind beneath your wings." Great, now I've got Bette Midler in my head. "It helps you want to care more about yourself and make better food choices," he told me. "You want to put better fuel in the tank."

Better fuel in the tank. Damn straight.

Sweet, Post-sweaty Dreams

Have you heard that loss of sleep makes you fat? In 2012, researchers from St. Luke's–Roosevelt Hospital and Columbia University presented to the American Academy of Sleep Medicine their fMRIs of 25 men and women showing that lack of sleep led to increased cravings for junk food.[22]

A number of other recent studies show a host of metabolic, hormonal and just plain old "too damn tired to exercise or eat properly" effects of insufficient sleep that lead to weight gain.[23]

And do you think there might be a few studies showing that exercise improves sleep? Yeah, there are; more than a few.[24]

THREE DANGEROUS WORDS

Don't blow it.

No, those three aren't the ones. But it's important to know that lots of people do all this hard work with exercise, reap tremendous brain benefits, and then they blow it.

Dr. Yoni Freedhoff believes that it's these three little words that can cripple all your weight loss efforts: "Because I exercised."

Yeah, this is the part where I tell you about how a lot of people screw this whole exercise thing up.

How Exercise Improves Eating Behavior

There is a lot to digest (lame pun—gak!) about how exercise affects eating, so here's a brief recap:

- Exercise reduces stress and helps alleviate depression, helping to control emotional eating.
- Exercise makes your brain fatigue-resistant, so it has the energy to think clearly about what you should eat. This is further enhanced by exercise improving quality of sleep.
- Exercise enhances the brain's executive function, improving your ability to stick to a healthy eating plan.
- Exercise—especially if it's intense—has an appetite-suppressing effect that can last for hours.
- On the psychological level, people who exercise regularly develop a keener interest in healthy eating to fuel their physical activities.

"There is a lot of evidence showing overweight people doing a little exercise and then overeating to compensate because they rationalize that they have earned themselves a reward," Eric Stice said.

Geez, a 2004 study of 94 people in *Appetite* found that just *reading* about exercise could cause people to eat more snacks.[25]

This is not the right way to think.

Here's the scenario: you've done all this exercise, which creates all these tremendous brain benefits revealed throughout this chapter—benefits that give you the *power to resist* junk food—and yet you can override those incredible effects by being stupid.

The "because I exercised" mentality is stupid. It's an illogical psychological breakdown for those looking to lose weight. If you feel that exercise isn't giving you the power to resist junk food, you might be overdoing it. You could be pushing so hard that you're causing a draining effect on your psyche. Instead of powering your brain to make wise food choices, you are—temporarily at least—robbing yourself of the energy to eat properly. It works on the same logic as sleep deprivation causing poor eating choices because you're too tired to make wise ones. So maybe you need to ease off on the physical activity. It's yet another reason why we advocate a slow and steady adoption of exercise to give both your body and your brain (and schedule) time to adapt.

The reward mentality—the bad math I mentioned where you think you've earned a 500-calorie piece of cheesecake after burning 300 calories on the treadmill—can be your downfall in all this. It's common. It's stupid, but it's common. THIS IS YOUR WARNING!

Don't do the reward mentality. Don't fall for this trap.

If you need to reward yourself, do it with fitness clothes, GPS gadgets, new running shoes, a massage or spa treatment. You can even reward yourself with a roll in the hay—anything but calories.

"The bottom line is that weight loss is 90 percent about diet," obesity researcher Dr. Sue Pedersen, a specialist in endocrinology and metabolism in Calgary, told me. "The studies show that exercise alone is not going to result in weight loss."

There are rare exceptions of people losing weight with just exercise, but for the vast majority you cannot out-exercise a bad diet. Again, think of exercise as your tool for better eating, not your excuse for lousy eating, because the calories burned via exercise can easily be undone (and then some) with one trip to the fast food drive-through.

Remember what Dr. Katz said: "You want to put better fuel in the tank."

Better fuel in the tank. Better fuel in the tank. Better fuel, better fuel . . .

STAGE II:
PREPARE

5

GET SMART:
METABOLISM MYTH BUSTING

Truth is so rare that it is delightful to tell it.

—EMILY DICKINSON

Welcome to Stage II, where the only sweating involves carrying shopping bags of fitness gear out to your car.

We're still in the "getting ready to get started" portion of your lifestyle overhaul. You've learned a lot about why junk food is so tempting, the reasons to change, and how exercise is your methadone for breaking highly palatable habits. Now it's time to "Prepare" before you "Do" the actual exercise and eating thing.

But start getting excited. Stage II involves building anticipation for awesome changes that will happen in Stage III. You may currently consider people who love working out and eating healthily to be insane; get ready to join the asylum.

An important part of preparation is shaking off the garbage that permeates Weight Loss Inc. and insinuates its way into your synapses. There are a lot of myths out there about how to lose weight, and exactly how much weight you can lose in how much time. As we've discussed, there is no money in marketing "slow and steady" to make the scale move, so most of what you've read and heard promotes an unrealistic mind-set.

Developing a sense of realism is an important part of the preparation process. It's time to shatter some delusions.

You're welcome.

THE MYTH OF RAPID WEIGHT LOSS

If you want to see a prime example of unrealistic weight loss expectations, look no further than the abysmal train-wreck fat-shaming TV game show *The Biggest Loser*, starring Jillian Michaels, who fancies herself "America's toughest trainer." In one of my articles, I called her on the "lose up to 5 pounds a week" weight loss claim she makes on her kettlebell DVD.

By the way, the kettlebell DVD wasn't the first time that Michaels had claimed you could lose up to five pounds a week. She had the same claim on her yoga DVD—you could lose almost a pound a day doing yoga. In other news, Snooki has been nominated for a Nobel in literature for *A Shore Thing*.

Let's get one thing straight: the only people who can lose a pound a day are the ones who start off weighing as much as a Smart car *and* are cattle-prodded by a team of sadists through a massive shift in lifestyle involving large amounts of exercise and significant dietary restriction. In other words: *not you*. And just because such people *can* lose weight that fast doesn't mean they should.

And yet, the ridiculous weight loss claims run rampant.

Fahren-hype 451

Go to the diet section of any bookstore and you'll see what I mean. I did *not* have to look hard to find these examples of fat-burning miracles.

"Drop up to 8 lbs in just 3 days!" This is taken straight from the cover of *The Belly Melt Diet,* from the editors of *Prevention.* This book claims MUFAs—monounsaturated fatty acids—have some kind of magic powers to, I don't know, change the molecular structure of belly fat and transport it to a parallel universe or something (Note: sarcasm). Either that or the book's pages are infected with amebic dysentery. That's the only way I know of to lose eight pounds in three days.

Here's another:

"Drop up to 14 lbs in the first 14 days." This one comes from *The Belly Fat Cure™ Fast Track,* by Jorge Cruise. You apparently achieve this amazingly rapid weight loss by discovering the "Ultimate Carb Swap™."

That's two trademark symbols on one cover. Must be because of all the extra awesome Jorge brings with that sexy name of his.

Some authors really like those words "up to," don't they? It's like their weight-loss-claim get-out-of-jail-free card. Hey, I GUARANTEE THAT WITH THIS BOOK YOU CAN LOSE *UP TO* ONE THOUSAND POUNDS THIS WEEK! See? I just made an outrageous promise and I can totally get away with it because I included "up to."

And that's not all.

If Jorge's "Fast Track" isn't fast enough, right next to it was his book *The Belly Fat Cure*™ (Again) *Sugar & Carb Counter*. It wants you to "Discover which foods will melt up to [those words again] 9 lbs. this week." Wait, so this one doesn't say "fast track," but it causes faster weight loss than the one that says "fast track"? I'm confused.

So are people who went to high school with Jorge, which might not be his sexy name after all. Back then his name was George Maurer.[1] Or was it Mauier?[2] I emailed him to ask which was the correct spelling, as well as to ask if he changed it because he thought the newer, sexier version would sell more books. Or was he, perhaps, in the witness protection program? He never got back to me. Anyway, I doubt that it's witness protection, because this guy likes going on *Oprah* and *Dr. Oz*, which isn't what I call low profile. With Oprah and Oz's help, George—or Jorge, or whatever—has sold over six million books and spent a lot of time on the *New York Times* best-seller list.

And just in case you don't read the weight loss claim in the starburst in the corner of the book's front cover, marketers have got you right there in the title now with *10 Pounds in 10 Days* by another *New York Times* best-selling author, Jackie Warner. The subtitle is *The Secret Celebrity Program for Losing Weight Fast*. I almost had an aneurysm from all those advertising buzzwords.

Just to be clear, we're talking about FAT loss here. I mean, you can achieve results like these via water loss (low-carb dieting can do that, by the way), but what's the point of just losing water? It comes right back.

Regarding burning fat, remember what we learned in chapter 2 about the first law of thermodynamics: calories are all that matter. For the average person, losing a pound a day requires running a marathon every 24 hours on a minuscule amount of food. That is neither reasonable nor sustainable. Speaking of sustained weight loss . . .

What Are the Odds?

Time for the most brutal honesty of the whole book: the odds are against you.

There are a wide variety of studies that look at people who are successful at *sustained* weight loss, and the results are not encouraging. On average, about 5 percent of people are successful at maintaining a significant drop in body weight, according to Dr. Arya Sharma, a professor of medicine and chair in obesity research and management at the University of Alberta.

Five percent? That sucks.

But wait! This 5 percent is representative of those who try every fad diet, miracle pill and exercise gimmick out there, and that is most people. In our efforts to get leaner, the majority of us are doing it wrong.

The National Weight Control Registry in the United States tracks several thousand people who have successfully maintained weight loss. The average amount lost is 66 pounds, and these people have kept it off for an average of 5.5 years.[3] Eighty-nine percent of these successful losers use a combination of diet and exercise. Walking is common, and on the diet side their strategies mostly involve cutting back on sugary and fatty foods. In other words, they take a logical and science-based approach to the whole thing.

And just FYI, 95 percent of them showed an improvement in quality of life—"a general measure of well-being that incorporates physical and psychological aspects," according to a 2009 report in *Medical Health Reviews.*[4]

So that's what people who are successful do. But what numbers do we have to show how many people will be successful when they eschew all the bogus gimmicks and take a thoughtful and effective approach to weight loss, like those in the Registry?

A group of researchers from respected medical institutions all over the US did a study of 5,145 obese men and women and published it in 2011 in the journal *Obesity*. These results are far more encouraging, but before I get into them, you should know that the participants qualify as tough cases. The average body weight put them into the second stage of obesity, and *all of them* had type 2 diabetes. The average weight for women was 209 pounds, and for men it was 240.

Yet even these tough cases had significantly improved success rates when their approach to weight loss involved paying attention to food intake, exercising and taking expert advice (i.e., not from Kim Kardashian).

After four years, almost a quarter of all the participants in the intervention group maintained a weight loss greater than 10 percent of their initial weight. Break the numbers down further and it gets even more encouraging. Some didn't do so well. Thirty-two percent lost almost nothing in the first year, and most of these people weren't that successful over the next three years either. It's a fact that a portion of the population won't succeed at weight loss no matter what. The fact that they didn't lose weight early on showed they were highly resistant to change. But what about those who did change?

Thirty percent lost about 8 percent of their body weight in year one (about 17 pounds for women and 19 pounds for men), and 40 percent of this group either maintained the weight loss over four years or kept on losing more.

The most aggressive losers fared the best. BUT the word "aggressive" does not mean TV's *The Biggest Loser*–style weight loss. Not even close. In the real world, "aggressive" translates to about 15 percent of starting body weight in year one. For the women in the study this meant an average of 31 pounds in a year; for men it was 36 pounds.

That's just over half a pound a week. And guess what happened? *Forty-two percent* of these people maintained greater than 15 percent weight loss through the four years of the study. What's more, an additional 28 percent sustained about half that amount of weight loss for four years.[5]

So you see, even if you qualify as a tough case, the numbers are far more encouraging when the right approach is taken.

Losing just over half a pound a week does indeed qualify as a tortoise pace. Even one pound a week is reasonable. Getting up to losing two pounds a week is at the outside of "reasonable."

Follow this plan and you've got a considerable chance at succeeding. There are no guarantees. We'll stack the deck in your favor the best we can by giving you the highest-quality information possible, but in the end it comes down to you.

I'm not talking about pounds when I say you're the one with the most to gain.

Now that we've dispelled some of the more blatant weight loss myths, it's time to get into the next stage of preparation: understanding how your metabolism works. We'll start with . . .

CALORIES OUT

You've likely seen infomercials for crappy plastic products or workout DVDs that talk about how much it's going to rev up your metabolism to *blast calories and incinerate fat!* Burning calories is peachy, but it's a small part of the overall equation that leads to lasting weight loss.

We're starting this chapter off discussing the calories you burn rather than the calories you ingest because it's the same order you're going to follow for the Virtuous Cycle. Exercise first, then diet.

That being said, I don't want you to sweat the numbers. Trying to figure out caloric balance, positive or negative, on a daily basis is an exercise in separating fly poop from pepper. You're about to find out the soul-crushingly depressing reasons why.

The purpose of this section is to give you an idea of how many calories some exercises burn so you can integrate this bit of knowledge into your lifestyle overhaul plan. Far more important will be gaining a "caloric awareness"—note, this is not the same thing as counting calories—of the food you eat, but we'll get to that in coming chapters.

Metabolism: The Basics

According to www.medterms.com, metabolism is "the whole range of biochemical processes that occur within us (or any living organism).

Metabolism consists both of anabolism and catabolism (the buildup and breakdown of substances, respectively). The term is commonly used to refer specifically to the breakdown of food and its transformation into energy."

In relation to weight loss, you are mostly concerned with that last sentence and the rate at which it takes place. In the simplest sense, the more work you put your body through, the more energy it requires to complete this work. If it doesn't get the energy it needs via food (because you're being careful about "calories in"), it will tap into fat stores to find this energy. "Tapping into fat stores" is good. That's what you want. If you're doing it wrong, you also lose muscle to compensate for this energy deficit, but exercise—especially resistance exercise like weightlifting—will ensure that muscle is preserved and it's fat that gets burned.

The Bad News

Getting in shape, restricting calories, losing weight: all these things *lower* your metabolism.

It's a bummer, but you can't escape it. Sure, you've been programmed by Weight Loss Inc. to believe there are miracle methods to boost your metabolism. After all, this type of claim sells books and drives clicks, and weight loss is a big cash business.

None of this makes the claims true.

Here are the basics of why:

- If you lose 50 pounds, that's 50 pounds less weight you carry with you everywhere you go. Every single activity becomes easier and requires less effort. This means fewer calories burned on a daily basis. It's simple logic.
- Having a lower body mass also lowers resting metabolism. There is less *you* requiring caloric expenditure to sustain various bodily functions.
- If you run a mile while in poor shape, you feel ready to barf up your toenails. Your heart is racing, lungs rasping, and you stay this way for a while afterward. This sensation of utter wretchedness

means you're burning lots of calories. Improve your physical condition, however, and running a mile becomes easy. You are more efficient. Your heart and lungs don't work as hard, and everything gets back to normal soon after you stop. You burn fewer calories. Also, recall the first point about how you might be carrying less weight on these runs as well.

Sorry, but the bad news about metabolism is just beginning.

How Eating Less Lowers Metabolism

When you eat less, your body burns fewer calories because its digestive system has less work to do.

"The calorie deficit decreases after the first day because energy expenditure starts to slow down immediately in regard to this restriction," explains Eric Ravussin, director of the Nutrition Obesity Research Center at Pennington Biomedical Research Center in Louisiana. "What is a 500 calorie deficit on day one is less so on day two, and even less on day three, and so on."

And it just keeps compounding. "By the 30th day of calorie restriction," Ravussin says, "what started off as a 500 calorie per day deficit has dropped to 300 or 250 calories per day."

In the strictest sense, the math of there being 3,500 calories in a pound of fat still holds true. However, sustaining that daily level of restricting 500 calories per day below maintenance level requires eating less and less each day to keep up with the drop in metabolism. This is because when you lose weight, "maintenance" keeps shifting downward. But continuing to cut calories more and more isn't a good idea either.

"If you are doing that," Ravussin says, "you're going to reach a level where you won't have all the essential nutrients for health."

Combating the Slowdown with Exercise

While metabolic slowdown can be combated with exercise, it's not a miracle cure. Claude Bouchard—an internationally renowned obesity researcher also at Pennington—led a series of studies in 1997 that provide interesting mathematical insight into caloric deficits.

In one study, seven pairs of male identical twins were kept on "no exercise" maintenance level calories. The researchers then added 1,000 calories of expenditure via stationary bicycling nine out of every 10 days for a 93-day period (a lot of exercise, for certain). They estimated that the participants created a 58,000 calorie deficit during the experiment, but the average weight loss—which was all from fat stores—represented the equivalent of only 46,000 calories.

The reverse happens too, as the team also experimented with 12 pairs of male twins, *adding* 1,000 calories of food over maintenance level for 100 days. Only 60 percent of these extra calories turned into weight gain. This is because metabolism goes up, but so do, uh, trips to the bathroom.[6]

In regard to the role of exercise, Ravussin sent me a study he co-wrote, published in June 2012 in the *Journal of Clinical Endocrinology and Metabolism*, which showed that even when vigorous exercise was included as part of a massive weight loss regimen for the severely obese in order to preserve fat-free mass, this "did not prevent dramatic slowing of resting metabolism."[7]

"It's much easier for obese people to cut 500 calories' worth of food than burn it off from running," he told me.

Yes, it's easier for the obese to cut food from a strictly caloric sense, but this does not discount the immense importance of exercise in weight loss, in case chapter 4 didn't drive that point home.

Diet alone to lose weight is a foolish idea. "There are autonomic, metabolic and hormonal reactions that make you regain. It's a whole body response," Dr. Alonso-Alonso said. "Physical activity is critical in terms of strengthening executive function to combat these physiological impulses to regain weight."

He's adamant. "Unless you pair diet with exercise, the weight is going to come back."

And if you incrementally push your limits, you can reach a point where exercise begins to make a significant contribution to caloric deficits. It just takes a fair bit of exercise.

Numbers Worth Knowing

As mentioned above, there are 3,500 calories in one pound of stored body fat. Also worth knowing is that one pound of body muscle contains about 600 calories *when used as fuel* (which is bad). However, because of a complex set of reactions, it takes *approximately* 2,500 calories to *build* a pound of muscle.

In order to burn off one pound of fat, you need to consume about 3,500 fewer calories than you burn. This is called creating a *caloric deficit*. Unlike in government budgets, a deficit is a good thing in the world of weight loss. If you were to look at the numbers over the course of a week, it would take an average daily deficit of about 500 calories to burn off a pound of fat.

Some *good* news is that weight training causes a portion (albeit a very small portion) of your caloric intake to turn into muscle, which helps in creating an overall negative energy balance (a caloric deficit). But since the majority of people gain muscle slowly (especially women), I wouldn't get too excited about calories getting partitioned toward muscle building if you're focusing on losing fat too.

The Easy Way to Calculate How Many Calories You Burn Each Day

Again, I'm not advocating obsessing over these numbers, because there is a lot of guesswork involved. That being said, there is still value in having a basic understanding of your individual caloric bank account in order to make wise decisions about how much to exercise and how much to eat.

So with the understanding that this is mostly guesswork, here's an easy way to determine how many calories you burn each day. Note that "easy" means "not that accurate." This method does not account for age or muscle mass (I'll provide a link to more accurate calculations later in this section). Here is how to get a rough idea:

- If you have a desk job and do little activity during the day, take your weight in pounds and multiply by 13 for men and by 12 for women.

- If your job is more active and/or you have to engage in some physical labor throughout the day, take your weight in pounds and multiply by 15 for men and by 14 for women.
- If you are moving for much of the day, engaged in a lot of non-exercise physical activity, then I'm wondering why you're reading this book. Still, if this is you, multiply your weight in pounds by 17 for men and by 16 for women.

An Important Measurement—Resting Metabolic Rate

Rough estimate again. To figure out your resting metabolic rate (RMR), take your weight in pounds and multiply by 10 if male or by 9 if female.

IMPORTANT: Then take that RMR number and divide by 24. Got it?

Me as an example: I weigh 170 pounds. Multiplied by 10 (remember, for women it's only multiplied by 9), that equals 1,700. Divide by 24 and you get 71. What does this "71" number mean? I'll tell you. It's how many calories I burn sitting on my butt every hour.

Knowing this allows you to calculate how many calories you burn *per hour* when you're *not* sitting on your butt.

It's about METs, or "metabolic equivalents." Your one-hour RMR calculation is 1 MET. Every time you get up and move around, the MET number climbs and you burn beyond your RMR. This is good. Here is a chart that shows an approximation of how many METs there are in various popular activities:

METs	Sport, Activity or Exercise
2.5	Slow walking, approximately 2 mph
3.0	Weightlifting: Light effort
3.0	Stationary bike: Very light effort
3.3	Walking at 3 mph
4.0	Water aerobics (aquacize)
5.0	Aerobic classes: Low impact
5.0	Walking at 4 mph
6.0	Weightlifting: Intense

7.0	Aerobic classes: High impact
7.0	Stationary bike: Moderate Effort
7.0	Swimming: Moderate effort
8.0	Circuit training, including aerobic stations, with no rest
8.0	Outdoor cycling at approximately 13 mph
9.0	Jogging at 5.2 mph (slow)
10.0	Outdoor cycling at approximately 15 mph
10.0	Running at 6 mph
10.0	Swimming fast
11.5	Running at 7 mph
13.5	Running at 8 mph
15.0	Running at 9 mph

Adapted from T. Baechle and R. Earle, eds., *Essentials of Strength Training and Conditioning*, 3rd ed. (Champaign, IL: Human Kinetics, 2008), 495–96.

There is a lot of guesswork when it comes to "calories out." Your definition of "intensity" plays a role, as does your level of coordination (a runner who looks as if he's got a scorpion in his underpants burns more calories than an efficient runner with a smooth gait), as well as other genetic and metabolic factors.

Subtraction: An Important Calculation

You know those 71 calories I burn each hour sitting around? If I do something to raise that amount, I need to take that 71 *away* from the total number to figure out the number of *extra* calories burned.

Me as an example again: As you learned, I burn about 71 calories per hour on the couch, but if I run for an hour at 6 mph (from the chart we know this elevates my metabolism to 10 METs), I burn a total of 710 calories during that hour. However, when thinking about how much caloric leeway this gives me, I need to remember that I would have burned 71 had I done nothing, so the *extra* calories are actually 710 minus 71, for a total of 639.

Don't Sweat the Numbers

You don't need to run these numbers. That's not my intent with this chart or these calculations. My intent is to build awareness. I want you to see how many extra calories certain activities burn so you know what type of impact they make in the overall weight loss equation.

In other words, understand that you need to exercise frequently—for long periods and at a high intensity—to have a profound impact on weight loss *from a calorie-burning perspective.*

I will repeat that the chart and RMR information are just to provide a reality check. They're to let you know that it takes a lot of exercise to wipe out even one treat. This entire section is about giving you perspective. Don't start adding up how many calories you've burned via exercise each day, because in most cases it just isn't going to help you lose weight. As you learned in chapter 4, it's important to remember that calorie burning is a distant second in importance to the positive brain changes resulting from exercise that transform you into a better eater.

Providing Caloric Leeway

Weight loss without exercise, beyond not giving you nearly as many health benefits, is so much harder that it seems insane not to make movement part of the program.

"Exercise ramps up your metabolism so that you don't need to go to such a low level of calories to lose weight," eating behaviorist Eric Stice told me. "You don't get into craving food. Exercise allows for more food to be eaten, which allows for better eating choices to be made because you're not ravenous." Again, you need to make sure that caloric balance is still negative in order to achieve weight loss and not get trapped in the reward mentality discussed in the previous chapter, but exercise gives you the ability to have more wiggle room so you're less likely to have those feelings of starvation that cause you to dive into a pile of salt-and-vinegar potato chips.

"Trying to lose weight without exercise is a horrible idea," Stice said. "You're setting yourself up to be tortured or to fail."

Shameless Self-promotion Alert!

I wrote a 13,000-word "Metabolism Report" (available free on my website) that boils down to repeating the advice in this section: essentially, "ignore your metabolism."

The report goes into excessive detail about how metabolism works, and then busts 12 of the most popular myths surrounding it.

Do you think that adding a bunch of muscle mass revs up your resting metabolism? Do you believe that interval training is the holy grail of fat loss? Do you think you should train in the "fat-burning zone," or exercise first thing in the morning on an empty stomach to "mobilize fat stores"?

If you answered yes to any of those questions, maybe you want to get the report. Did I mention it's free?

Go to my website, www.BodyForWife.com, and click on the Free Report link. You'll find other useful (and free) stuff on there as well, including easy-to-make, healthy, low-calorie dinner recipes by registered dietitian Lindy Kennedy and her students. They're free too.

Starting slowly with exercise is not just fine, it's what we recommend. Just remember that gradual and constant progression is important. It's not just more calories burned but a stronger will for dealing with food, not to mention an enhanced training response that sculpts your physique and makes you more physically capable and healthier from head to toe.

CALORIES IN

I knew a woman who had to eat a pint of Häagen-Dazs every day to keep from wasting away. Mind you, she was on the Olympic rowing team and training hard for more than 20 hours a week. At the end of each day she reached her limit of healthy "food as fuel" she could cram into her belly to fuel exercise, and the only thing she could mentally tolerate to sustain her weight was a bucket of ice cream. I like the kind with cookie dough.

If you're training hard for a grueling Olympic event, you get a lot of leeway in the calorie consumption department. Otherwise, you need to watch the "calories in" side of the weight loss equation to lose or maintain body weight.

Last summer we were on the coast at my parents' condo for three weeks. Each week I ran 35 miles, spent several hours in a sea kayak, swam a few miles and played a lot with my kids in the water. And I still gained weight.

In the condo we had three good cooks, and we all took turns preparing meals, trying to outdo each other with a gluttonous feast. There were fancy restaurant meals as well. Plus, it was vacation, so . . . booze.

Even using my vacation as if I were training for competition, I saw the little lines outlining my *rectus abdominis* disappear. I literally could not outrun all the food and beer.

Macronutrient Myths and Misinformation

Remember Twinkie Guy from chapter 2?

You can eat bacon-stuffed Froot Loops and lose weight if calories are negative. You can eat broccoli wrapped in spinach and gain weight if you manage to stuff in enough to make calories positive.

Paleo, wheat bellies, Atkins, gluten, saturated fat, sugar, insulin . . . the only thing that matters to *weight loss* is calories. Of course, there is weight loss and then there is healthy, sustainable fat loss. We advise the latter because it's better for you, and it creates a higher-performing and nicer-looking body.

We advocate a diet that maximizes health, keeps calories in check, is satisfying, sustainable and tastes good. Hmmm . . . that seems kind of important. Let's highlight this.

Your diet should

- Maximize health
- Keep calories in check
- Be satisfying
- Be sustainable
- Taste good

On that last point, remember the mango versus carrot cake argument. There's a big difference between "good" and "unnatural taste-bud-explosion amazeballs."

The problem with so many diets is that they often ignore any or all of these common-sense diet traits in pursuit of some gimmick. Remember the rejection letter at the beginning of this book? Remember that whole Weight Loss Inc. thing I mentioned? Sensationalism sells.

The snake oil salesman is alive and well, and he's still in the health and fitness business.

Screw that guy.

Reaching Out to Real Experts

One thing I've noticed about writers and bloggers for gimmicky diets is that they have a tendency to cherry-pick and misinterpret research. I could load this section with references, and people with either irrelevant credentials or no credentials at all would counter with twisted viewpoints to defend their positions (and their profits). Some embrace low-carbohydrate dieting with fundamentalist zeal and feel compelled to smite grain-eating infidels. This is unlike vegans, who never proselytize or guilt-trip anyone about the evils of animal holocaust.

The hate mail for this book is going to be epic.

So instead of loading up the endnotes, I decided to talk to smart people with relevant and respected credentials and a proven track record of helping people achieve realistic and lasting weight loss (and enhanced physical performance). Is this an appeal to authority? I trust the opinions of these experts far more than the advice of some guy who runs a blog that's jam-packed with ads for low-carb products. That's why I had the content of this book vetted by a registered dietitian who has consulted face to face with thousands of real clients.

My adviser is Lindy Kennedy; in addition to being a registered dietitian (RD) she has a master's of science in health promotion. I found Lindy because I heard her on the radio. She sounded smart, so I Google-stalked her. And she *is* smart, and science-based. Most RDs are.

Why am I telling you this? You may need extra nutritional coaching beyond this book. In fact, I support your finding a respected registered dietitian to consult on your diet. They're not all perfect. Some have gone to the dark side, but in my experience the majority of them are solid.

Be wary of anyone calling him- or herself a "holistic nutritionist," because it's an unaccredited designation that embraces alternative, pseudoscientific ideas about nutrition. Also, they love flogging supplements.

With so many quacktacular diet gurus out there extolling their way as the best way, it can be hard to separate fact from fiction. One way to help identify nutritional nonsense is to know that . . .

Truth Is Not a One-liner

"We have a lot of different people demonizing different things," Dr. David Katz told me. "They're falling in love with their own hypotheses. Sugar! Eggs! Protein! Carbs! A lot of this is an attempt to sell something, but the challenge with the truth is that it is not a one-liner. It's not just to avoid carbs. These people are salesmen, and one-liners can make you rich."

They sure made Pierre Dukan, author of *The Dukan Diet*, wealthy. His book was just another form of low-carb dieting, and unless you count Suzanne Collins's *The Hunger Games*, Dukan's is the best-selling diet book of all time, with 10 million copies sold. His diet has sold as many copies as *Catch-22*, *A Brief History of Time*, *The Cat in the Hat* and *The Joy of Sex*.

Excuse me while I go kill myself.

Well, my wife is a physician who makes a good salary, so I can tell you the truth and not have to subsist on cat food in my retirement. Don't worry about me; I'll be fine. Especially if I can get the future Queen of England to follow our program the way she did Pierre Dukan's.

Another thing worth knowing when it comes to designing your new diet is that . . .

Wheat ≠ Satan

I asked sport nutrition expert and registered dietitian Nancy Clark about the demonization of wheat in books lately, and she said, "I've gone through the demonization of fat, meat, eggs and nuts. This is just one more on the list. What will they think of next? I am not jumping on that bandwagon."

Regarding the latest anti-gluten craze, Clark explained that celiac disease affects less than 1 percent of the population, and about 6 percent of the population is gluten intolerant. "But that means 93 percent can enjoy it just fine."

And yet we have neurologist Dr. David Perlmutter making the statement "Gluten is this generation's tobacco."[8] The ridiculousness of this comparison boggles the mind. Only 1 percent of the population is celiac, and yet according to the World Health Organization tobacco kills 50 percent of its regular users.[9] Could it be Dr. Perlmutter has a carbohydrate-vilifying book to sell? Yup. It's called *Grain Brain*. After the success of *Wheat Belly* the bandwagon just keeps on a-rolling. What's the next grain-based boogeyman? Rye thigh? Oat bloat?

Clark says anecdotal reports of people feeling better when they ditch wheat are easily explained. "When they go off wheat, it means no burgers . . . or cookies or doughnuts, so of course they're going to feel better." An excellent resource I recommend to all active people is *Nancy Clark's Sport Nutrition Guidebook*. It's a book about fueling exercise, an approach that promotes weight loss.

I'm going bromance on you about Alan Aragon. He has a master's of science in nutrition and is sought out by organizations such as the L.A. Lakers, L.A. Kings and Anaheim Mighty Ducks as well as Olympians, physique competitors and average folks looking for nutrition advice. I've read a ton of his stuff and interviewed him for a number of articles. When it comes to separating nutritional fact from fiction, I trust him more than most.

I specifically asked Alan about the book *Wheat Belly* and the current vilification of grains.

"I think it's silly," he said. "There is no consistent evidence that wheat is bad. There's a small percentage of people who are gluten intolerant," he said, echoing Clark. "The overwhelming majority can include wheat-based foods and live a good and healthy life. It's the consumption of the highly refined stuff that's a problem." Grains need to contribute to a caloric surplus for them to be a bad thing, he said.

Aragon also said the paleo diet—a form of low-carb dieting that its advocates presume our Stone Age, hunter-gatherer ancestors ate—is just another fad. "Paleo philosophy is wrong on a couple of different levels," he told me. "They say our ancestors didn't eat grains, and therefore we shouldn't eat grains. First, our ancestors *did* eat grains. There is also the logical error that if our ancestors didn't eat something, we shouldn't either. Well, our ancestors didn't concern themselves with optimal nutrition, they just wanted to survive.

"It's just another fad," Clark said, echoing Aragon's opinions on paleo. "There's no science to support it."

Aragon told me that vilifying any food group misses the big picture. He also attacks those who believe sugar is toxic. "They have no sense of moderation," Aragon told me. "They err on philosophical levels and on the scientific level. They're up in arms about fructose being toxic, and the studies they reference showing fructose is a problem are [based on the consumption of] three times what the average American takes in."

"Active people can tolerate sugar much better than couch potatoes," Nancy Clark said. This supports Mayo Clinic's Dr. Joyner's statement in chapter 3 about exercise trumping a lot of bad behaviors.

"You can push anything to extremes and get abnormal responses," Richard Mattes, a registered dietitian and distinguished professor of nutrition at Purdue University in Indiana, told me. "There are limits to what people choose to do."

Yes, you can still have your treats. I'll remind you that this is not an all-or-none approach. Make your indulgences less frequent and because you really want them. Pick something tasty and make it worth the calories.

The major lesson here is that "macronutrient mixture (protein, carbohydrates, fat) is not predictive of weight loss or gain," Mattes said. "Total calories are the common denominator." Again, it always boils down to calories.

Fat Is Misunderstood

I often read about the latest diet craze and shake my head. Some push a diet that is 50 percent fat. Well, there's a good reason not to eat so much fat, so let's start there.

First off, know that not all macronutrients are created equal. Let's break them down in chart form:

	Fat	Carbohydrates	Protein
Calories per gram	9	4	4
Effect on satiety	Low	Moderate	High
Thermic effect	Low	Moderate	High

Look at that first column. Fat has more than twice as many calories per gram as either protein or carbohydrates. This means that when something contains a lot of fat, it translates to a massive amount of extra calories jammed into a small volume of food. Fat is also low for satisfying appetite, and low for "thermic effect," which means it burns almost none of its own calories during the process of digestion.

Protein, conversely, burns off about 20 percent of its calories just being digested. Don't let this tempt you to go high protein, however, because when you run the numbers, it doesn't make a significant difference. (See the Metabolism Report available on my website for more details.)

Much of the negative hype over the health effects of certain saturated fats has been overblown. Dr. Katz told me that when new research came out, he went back to eating eggs. I eat eggs too. Lots of them. What's more, "there are a lot of interesting studies showing that dairy saturated fat doesn't lead to earlier death," Nancy Clark said. "The fat in cheese, milk and butter doesn't raise cholesterol. However, if you're trying to lose weight, it's the fatty foods you want to watch out for because they easily turn into body fat."

There is also the fact that fat makes things taste good, as explained in chapter 2, potentially leading to overconsumption.

There are certain levels of all three macronutrients needed for optimal health and performance. Demonizing any one of them is stupid, and often profitable if you're a "diet guru."

How Much of What?

So fine, you're saying. I need a bit of everything. But how do I know how much of what? How much of which macronutrient you need is somewhat dependent on activity level. The quick explanation is this: more exercise = more carbohydrates.

"There is not a lot of extra room for carbs when training volume is low," Alan Aragon said. "When you're cutting calories for weight loss, carbs are going to have to bear the brunt of the restriction because you can't cut too far into protein or fat or you'll lose muscle and inhibit certain hormone functions." It's important to note the point about "when training volume is low." That means this applies only to people who barely exercise.

Focusing on Good Fats

For a person who isn't that active, Aragon says a good minimum for fat intake is about 20 percent of total calories. Not 50 percent but 20 percent. He also stated that it's safer for women to go lower in fat than men because it's testosterone that's affected the most by decreased fat intake, and men need that more.

"When people restrict fat too much, they miss out on the health-promoting and disease-preventing aspects of healthy fats." These healthy fats are found in things such as nuts, seeds, avocados, olives, peanut butter and fatty fish such as salmon, tuna, mackerel, herring, trout and sardines.

Trans fats, which high-processed junk food is full of, are the main things to avoid. Saturated fats from dairy and eggs are okay but should be limited from meats.

Protein by the Numbers

Aragon advocates protein intake between 0.7 and 1 gram per pound of body weight per day, if you don't mind mixing metric and imperial measurements. For me, at 170 pounds, that's between 120 and 170 grams of protein a day. With protein checking in at 4 calories per gram, I need to take in *at most* 680 calories' worth of protein a day, which isn't a lot, to *gain* more muscle. Oh, and protein doesn't always mean "meat." Besides eggs and dairy, there are plenty of plant-based ways to get it, such as beans, nuts, seeds, whole grains and oats, peas, lentils, and vegetables such as avocados, broccoli, spinach and sweet potato.

Nancy Clark is a little more restrained in her protein recommendations: "The RDA [recommended dietary allowance] for the average person is 0.4 grams per pound of body weight. For an active person I recommend 0.5 to 0.75 grams per pound." Clark also stated that she is an advocate of dairy. "I think it's really high-quality nutrition," she said. I agree. Milk is my post-exercise recovery drink.

And since we're on the subject of recovery drinks, don't go believing you need protein supplements. If you're juiced to the gills on anabolic steroids and lifting as if your life depends on it to pack on enough muscle mass to resemble some kind of goalie-mask-wearing *Road Warrior* bad guy, then go for it. For the rest of us, including the dedicated weightlifters wanting to build an esthetically pleasing level of muscle, your protein needs can be met via real food without difficulty. There could be exceptions for vegans, so if you are one, consult an RD.

Good Carbs, Bad Carbs

As I mentioned earlier, more exercise means more carbohydrates. There's ample evidence that carbs are the best source of fuel for activity. I feel as though my body craves them. But they've got to be the good kind. The refined sugars and grains—the junk food and chips and white bread and soda and all that other garbage—is to be avoided. But the healthy kind is great fuel. Whole-wheat whole-grain bread, bagels and pasta are nutrient-dense rocket-fuel go juice for exercise. Fruits and vegetables are awesome for health, satiety and physical performance. (We'll explain how to know the difference between good carbohydrates and bad ones in coming chapters.)

Alan Aragon says that a low-carbohydrate diet can be good for some people, but it's not a good choice for a physically active person, and considering the exercise recommendations of this book, it is not a dietary method we advocate.

"One merit of low carb, if you can call it a merit," Aragon stated, "is a simplification of diet. It becomes easier to remember and to stick to." Going low carb does mean cutting Froot Loops, so that part is good, at least. Personally, I'm a big fan of going low *refined* carb.

What Is a Good Diet?

"Michael Pollan's advice is pretty darn good," Dr. Katz told me, referencing the author's advice: "Eat food. Not too much. Mostly plants."[10]

That "eat food" part? Katz explained that Pollan is referring to things with a short ingredient list. For example, an apple contains . . . one apple. That makes it a good choice. That makes it food. An ingredient list that looks as if someone loaded three dozen keyboards into a 12-gauge shotgun and blasted it at the label is not food. It is not a good choice.

The keyboard-shotgun-label stuff makes highly palatable food. But it's humans messing with nature and adding a bunch of unspeakable crap to override your taste buds and create out-of-control consumption. We want you to stop eating so much of that stuff.

So, yeah. Eat food. And our experts don't want you to fall for the paleo mentality suggesting that you can live off mammoth meat or something. Remember: mostly plants.

You Decide How Much "Food" and How Many Plants

Although Katz advocates Pollan's three simple rules as a good starting mantra, he also pointed me to an article of his own called "Separation of Church and Plate."[11]

In it, he describes how some foods, like bread, can be processed and are still okay. Even meat that's been cooked is processed. A short ingredient list doesn't mean only one ingredient. The whole-wheat whole-grain bread I eat has a number of ingredients, and most of them are good. The not-so-good ones are few and in small quantities.

Katz wants us to avoid religious fervor about food. Just understand what is good, and shoot for getting as close to that as you can manage without life sucking or you needing to develop an obsessive-compulsive disorder over what you eat.

Another Katz article had this question as its title: "Can We Say What Diet Is 'Best'?" And the answer is no, we don't know what is best.

"And anyone who claims we know decisively what specific diet is best for health is either misguided, selling something or both,"[12] Katz writes. He advocates a *theme* of healthy eating that emphasizes fruits and vegetables, whole grains, beans and nuts.

I will say it again and again: this isn't all or none. Do your best, and incrementally try to improve your diet. Find something you can enjoy and sustain. And if you need additional help, find a reputable registered dietitian to consult.

Encouraging Intelligent Feedback

I know I'll get more candidates for my "Intelligent Feedback" email folder because of this.

Exercise is a critical part of this program, and low-carb diets aren't so good for enhancing physical performance. I'll do another one of those mega endnotes supporting diets that are high in unrefined carbohydrates for exercise performance.[13] What's more, I've interviewed numerous Olympic champions, and without exception they all extol the virtues of carbs for exercise fuel. Remember, we're creating a Virtuous Cycle with exercise and healthy eating reinforcing each other. Demonizing a food group that fuels exercise is stupid.

Low-carb can work okay for people on low or no exercise, but you can aspire to better than that. You can aspire to not just losing weight but being physically fit. Lindy, Margaret and I think low-carb dieting is a half-assed way to lose weight.

Our way is better, so choose our way. Choose full-assed.

6

GET REAL: CHANGING HOW YOU VIEW FOOD

One should eat to live, not live to eat.

—BENJAMIN FRANKLIN

Lean bodies are made in the kitchen.

You *need* food, and an appropriate amount of it, especially to fuel exercise. Starvation is not the way to go about this. When you learn to love food that loves you back, your appetite is easier to control, you're energized, you feel better, and weight comes off. But before you start choosing those foods, we need to do a little more myth busting, because what you see on TV is what sells, not what's actually true.

I've seen infomercials spouting, "Eat whatever you want! Eat as much as you want!" They make me want to punch my TV, and I love my TV.

The reality is this: to lose weight, you get to do neither. Well, if you focus on eating mostly healthy food—food that is good but doesn't have such an amazing flavor that your taste buds go into overdrive—you will be able to get close to eating as much as you want, because healthy food does a better job of filling you up. More important, it doesn't cause satiety signals in the body and brain to malfunction so that you keep shoveling it in faster than Rush Limbaugh and Michael Moore going through a shared plate of chicken wings.

LOVE FOOD THAT LOVES YOU BACK

"You need to love food that loves you back," Dr. Katz told me.

Food that loves you back is food that tastes good, is filling, healthy, fuels physical activity and doesn't cause you to overeat. Food that does *not* love you back has been manufactured to taste unnaturally good. It's not filling, not healthy and you can't control intake. Our approach is about focusing more on the former and much less on the latter.

Slim and fit people are not those who see food as a source of constant indulgence. To "indulge" is to give in to one's desires. If you do it all the time, it begins to lose its meaning. It's no longer an indulgence or a treat but a way of life—a way of life that's a leading cause of obesity.

I am not made of stone. I derive great pleasure from inhaling an extra-cheese-laden Hawaiian pizza chased with a beer or four while gluing my butt to the couch to watch some high-definition violence on my 52-inch LCD screen. But if I were to do this every day, it would lose its value as an indulgence; it would become the norm. Also, I'd be fat.

Treat foods need to become just that: a treat to be enjoyed—savored—on occasion, rather than a primary source of fuel and nutrition.

Focus on Foods That Fill

I'll teach you a trick right now. It's called "Can I eat an apple?"

First off, apples go in the fridge. I've had apples last for months in there. Buy a bag of the kind you like (feel free to mix them up) and make sure you've always got apples on hand. Bring at least one to work each day. You could even get a plastic container, decorate it with your name and pictures of skulls and crossbones, maybe slap on a padlock, and put it in the community fridge. You can write "contains apples" on the container too; your co-workers will look at it and say, "Meh, not worth stealing."

So, yeah, have apples on hand. And when you feel the need to snack, ask yourself the question. Did you forget the question? The question is, can I eat an apple? If the answer is no, you are not hungry enough to eat a snack. Of course, it's not going to work every time. If there are Boston cream doughnuts in a meeting, I *will* eat one. Those things are awesome.

But that simple question can make you stop. It can make you think. It can make you decide you don't need a snack. Alternatively, it can make you say, "Hell, yeah. An apple sounds great right now." And then you eat one. Apples don't have many calories, are filling and you rarely want more than one.

Unlike doughnuts.

If the doughnut/apple thing isn't clear enough for you, here's an even more extreme example of filling versus non-filling foods. My grocery store sells big plastic tubs of fresh baby spinach. These tubs are twelve inches long by seven inches wide by three inches deep. One tub contains 11 ounces of spinach. That's more than two-thirds of a pound. The number of calories it contains is less than what is in a single Oreo cookie.

I don't know how many tubs of spinach I can eat in one sitting (I've never tried), but I can sure eat more than one Oreo.

Some researchers believe the caloric density of food is paramount when it comes to satiety. This Oreo-spinach example may lead you to believe the same. The Oreo is calorically dense; it packs a massive wallop of calories in a small volume of food. Uh, I mean "food." The spinach, on the other hand, is low in caloric density: big volume of food, not many calories.

But there's more to satiety than that. As Dr. Katz said, "Truth is not a one-liner." Yes, volume is important. Taking in a great volume of food for few calories can help you feel full; a number of studies have shown this.[1] However, this fact coincides with the fact that food low in caloric density is often healthier and lower in reward value too. Calorically dense foods, like Oreos, are sugar-fat-crap sandwiches that overwhelm taste buds and promote runaway pie-hole shoveling.

"Energy density is a popular concept," Purdue University nutrition professor Richard Mattes told me. "But it's one dimension of food. You can eat a larger volume of food for the same or fewer calories, but the problem is that you don't eat vegetables whole; chewing makes them smaller." Seeing a big volume of food on the plate can have a cognitive effect on satiety as well, Mattes explained. Seeing that much food is going to make you think it's more filling, but chewing evens things out a bit.

Choosing Wisely at the Macro Level

Let's reaffirm the information from the chart in chapter 5.

I consulted Raylene Reimer, a registered dietitian and associate professor of nutrition and metabolism at the University of Calgary. "Protein has the highest satiety factor of the three macronutrients, carbohydrates come second, and fat is hardly satiating at all," she told me.

Richard Mattes said the same thing, but added, "Protein in solid food is good, but in liquid form it doesn't seem to retain its superiority in terms of being satiating." He explained that when people, such as the elderly, are having trouble keeping weight on, protein shakes like Ensure are often used to provide extra calories.

Shaking Things Up

And then Mattes and I had a little segue into weight loss shakes.

"Shakes for weight loss work by portion control," he said. They create a set of rules. If you buy a "weight loss shake," it "works" by getting you to follow certain rules to lower total daily caloric intake. Slim-Fast used the line, "A shake for breakfast, a shake for lunch, then a sensible dinner." If one can of Slim-Fast has 220 calories, breakfast and lunch total only 440 calories. If by some miracle you're *not* starving at dinnertime and can stick to that "sensible dinner" plan, then yes, these simple rules can allow for a calorie-restricted diet that will lead to weight loss. There's nothing miraculous about the shake. It possesses no magic fat-burning properties. It's not satiating, and it sure isn't as healthy as a balanced diet.

And it isn't sustainable either. You may be able to stick to a plan like this for a while via white-knuckle starvation, but at some point your hunger will get the better of you, and then Old Country Buffet, here you come.

There's a reason why professional bodybuilders use protein shakes— it's to jam in the *extra calories* needed to build ridiculous amounts of muscle. As a weight loss tool, the use of shakes is foolish. These things are meant for *weight gain*.

Blown Out of Proportion?

Solid protein and fiber are satiating. This fact has been a staple of weight loss advice for ages. But just *how* satiating are they?

"I think a lot of these truths that we've held about satiety have been overblown," Richard Mattes told me. "Foods are more than unidimensional. [Focusing solely on satiety] ignores the nutrient contribution a food might provide. Almonds are high in energy density but are a great source of vitamin E." See? High caloric density does not always equal bad.

"I think a diet somewhat higher in protein is probably useful," he said, "but it's not as dramatic and reliable as some believe. It's often overestimated." Mattes said the same of fiber. "It's been a workhorse of satiety for a long time. Depending on the fiber, it can lead to prolonged digestion and a better satiety response." He told me, however, that a lot of the study trials asserting the satiating effects of fiber use levels beyond what most people would be willing to eat. Still, "I would favor a diet that is high in fiber," he said. "It does have many other benefits, but the expectation that it will have a marked effect on appetite may be overestimated."

Multilevel Shake Marketing

I'm going to lose Facebook friends over this.

If you see people talking about how awesome a certain weight loss shake is, be it on Facebook or in person, you may want to think *Amway*. These folks may be part of a multilevel marketing (MLM) program. People call themselves a "Beach Body Coach" and flog the scientific-sounding "Shakeology." ViSalus shakes are another product sold via MLM, connected with something called "Body by Vi," and another shake is "IsaLean," also sold via MLM, by a company called Isagenix.

All those wonderful endorsements by your friends of how awesome these shakes are for weight loss? It could be that they're trying to sell them to you.

Things I have seen posted on Facebook:

- "17 pounds down! Thank you, ViSalus!"
- "Getting my Shakeology on! This is the best weight loss tool EVER!"
- "[Isagenix] transformed my life beyond my expectations."

A healthy diet, especially the kind that leads to weight loss, does not come in shake form.

LAY OFF THE LIQUID LUCIFER

Wheat is not the Devil, but soda sure as hell is. Let's call it Liquid Lucifer because I love alliteration.

Six percent of the calories that North Americans ingest are sugar-sweetened beverages. Add another 5 percent in booze calories for adults. These things (and this includes juice) do not satiate *at all*. A 2006 study published in the *Journal of the American Dietetic Association* found that when people drank water as opposed to juice, or diet soda as opposed to sugared soda, with a meal, the total *food* calories consumed in the meal was the same. In other words, all those extra calories in the juice and soda versus the water and diet soda did not have any impact on how many food calories these people ate. Instead, the juice and soda just added to total calories.[2] That's bad.

Juice does have health properties, but calories are high and satiety is low; for someone looking to lose weight, juice is a terrible choice. Oranges and apples and grapes are filling; orange juice and apple juice and grape juice are not. What's more, the juice versions add in a processing factor that removes things like fiber.

"I really do believe beverages are especially problematic," Mattes said. "They don't displace other energy sources. When you drink calories, it just adds to total energy."

And don't forget about high-calorie coffee drinks. Don't load in tons of cream and sugar, and never order those frappa-zappa-what-the-mocha-hella concoctions. They can have as many calories as a Big Mac. If you're skeptical, consider googling the calories of your favorite coffee drink. Prepare for a shock.

I do find skim milk to be good in moderation, however, especially right after exercise because it offers a rapid absorption of both carbohydrates and protein—macronutrients that a post-exercise body is in need of—and choosing the non-fat variety means calories are reasonable.

EMBRACE THE NORMAN ROCKWELL DIET

You know that Norman Rockwell painting of the family all sitting around the dinner table? You need to do more of that. Also, you need to do much less of *not that*.

I mean, eat meals at the family dinner table, and try not to eat meals that aren't at this table.

"My advice would be three to four meals a day and no more," Margriet Westerterp, a nutrition professor at Maastricht University in the Netherlands, told me. "Those should be real meals." Real meals mean sitting at a table, on a regular time schedule. And she advocates keeping snacking to a minimum.

In Canada, those living in the province of Quebec are the least likely to be overweight or obese in the entire country, and yet they eat far more desserts than in any other province.[3] The reason is that they are more like their European counterparts than their North American counterparts in that they don't embrace our snacking culture. They sit down to proper meals with higher regularity, and these meals do include dessert more often than those of Anglo families do. However, it's in the other provinces where we're snacking all the time. Constant snacking is what leads to higher caloric intake. If you're not snacking and are eating proper meals on a regular schedule, there's room, caloric-deficit speaking, for dessert more often.

The critical part to remember here is not so much that snacking is bad but that what we have a tendency to eat when we snack is often bad. Healthy snacks are good, but most of us don't eat healthy snacks. Apples and carrots sticks and unsalted nuts and sugar-snap peas, etcetera, are fine, but when you're reaching for the chips and doughnuts and chocolate, it's a problem.

And snacking throughout the day isn't our only downfall—nighttime can be particularly problematic. France Bellisle is a food intake behavior researcher in Paris. In 2004 she had an article published in the *Scandinavian Journal of Nutrition* titled "Impact of the Daily Meal Pattern on Energy Balance." In it she reported, "Obese people tend to eat little in the morning and much in the afternoon and evening. In extreme cases, a 'night-eating syndrome' is observed."[4]

Bellisle also attacks the notion of "six small meals a day" that was popularized by Bill Phillips in *Body for Life*.[5] Bellisle writes, "The notion [of greater meal frequency] has been put into question by the recognition of a high level of dietary underreporting in overweight individuals.

In addition, no difference in total daily energy expenditure has been documented as a function of daily meal number. Weight loss is not facilitated by high meal frequency. Snacking in obese subjects is associated with higher energy and fat intake."[6]

Snacking often means you're not paying attention to what you're eating. It means you're eating frequently and it's hard to keep track of intake. It also means you're more prone to food cues and high-calorie treats. Changing your views so you see eating as something that happens at the dinner table on a regular schedule means that you're well fueled throughout the day. You eat less because you're not so likely to fall prey to the temptation to snack.

Nancy Clark likes four meals a day: breakfast, lunch, second lunch and dinner. "The purpose of second lunch is to not overeat at dinner." Lindy Kennedy likes this mini lunch around three in the afternoon as well.

Tips for Cutting Down on Snacking

We've shown that Western culture is a junk food snacking culture, and this makes us fat. You now know the importance of real meals at scheduled times around the dinner table, and this involves a decrease in snacking to be effective. Here are tips to reduce the temptation to snack:

- As soon as you get home from work, take a shower. We don't actually want you to waste water, but when it comes to snacking, a shower can be an extra-effective deterrent. Many of us go straight to the fridge after work. If you head for the shower instead of the kitchen, you're getting naked and doing something rewarding. If you're worried about hair and makeup, just focus on areas from the neck down. It will still feel good. It doesn't have to be a long shower, and you can change into some comfortable clothes afterward.
- Chew some sugarless gum.
- Ask yourself the apple question. If the answer is yes, eat an apple. If the answer is no, don't eat at all.
- Avoid locations where snacks are present. Don't walk past places where they are sitting out and tempting you. Pay for gas at the

pump rather than going into the store. Stay away from aisles in stores loaded with snacks.

- Keep pistachios on hand for times when the temptation to snack hits. They're among the lowest-calorie nuts, and you need two hands to crack the shells. After less than a dozen you start thinking, *Uh, I have things to do. I can't be using both hands for this long just to eat.*
- Buy peeled and washed carrots and keep some in a bowl of water in the fridge. Reach for those instead.
- Don't have high-calorie snacks in the house. If you live with other people who enjoy such snacks, you have a couple of options. One is to get them on board with your eating program; another is to ask them to hide such snacks from you, or to choose snacks you don't like. When shopping for cookies for the kids, I purposely purchase ones I'm not fond of.

AVOID THE STARVATION RESPONSE

Seriously cutting back calories (below about 1,500 per day for a man and below 1,200 per day for a woman) day after day can cause a significant metabolic slowdown. Several days of moderate to moderately high caloric deficits, and even the occasional short fast, *are not* going to cause a starvation response, especially if your caloric deficits are at least in part attributed to adding in a bunch of physical activity.

What is this "starvation response"? Back in the 1940s, when people were more tolerant of being guinea pigs, nutrition researchers at the University of Minnesota Ancel Keys conducted the Minnesota Starvation Study (actually, the participants were conscientious objectors to World War II). Thirty-six men were subjected to an extended period of 50 percent of their maintenance-level caloric needs (the purpose was to learn about how to·deal medically with impending starvation as a result of the war—it wasn't just a lark). As a result of participation, the men's metabolic rates dropped a substantial amount, in part due to loss of body mass but also due to an evolutionary advantage that results in the body using fewer calories during lean times.[7]

The starvation response doesn't sound like much of an advantage these days, but back when the hunt failed or there was a drought, it sure came in handy: it kept people alive. Another metabolic response programmed in by natural selection is "post-starvation hyperphagia." I asked my wife (the doctor) what hyperphagia meant, and she replied, "Pigging out."

After they've experienced a period of starvation, a hormonal response causes people to overeat past what it takes to replace the lost weight, gaining more than they lost in the first place. In the bad old days this extra fat protected them against the next time food was in short supply, but today it just causes yoyo dieting, with the dieters ending up fatter than when they started.[8]

So how do you prevent starvation response?

Don't cut calories too much. An average-sized man (weighing around 180 pounds) should consume a minimum of 1,800 calories per day, and the average woman 1,400. Note that these are estimates and will vary based on body size.

The bare minimum I eat on a daily basis is about 2,000 calories, except for this one day after a draft beer bender when I felt like, uh, never mind. On a day that I don't exercise, I burn about 2,200 calories. But I do exercise most days of the week. A lot. So I'm usually eating significantly more than that 2,000 calorie minimum.

Also, don't restrict calories every single day. Take one day a week when you break even or go a little over. *But do not* use your "binge" day to go nuts. You can wipe out three or four days of caloric deficits in one day of runaway gluttony. Not restricting calories once a week is about the psychological benefits of not feeling deprived. If you're being careful, you can have caloric deficits every single day as long as it's not making you crazy. Having a day when you go over a little isn't critical to preventing starvation response. Remember that starvation response comes from actually starving yourself, not from cutting calories wisely.

"I recommend that people go 10 to 20 percent below maintenance calories to lose weight," Nancy Clark said. "Cutting calories in half is not sustainable. It leads to rebound overeating and yoyo dieting."

If you need to take in 2,000 calories to stay at your current weight, cutting down to the 1,600 to 1,800 range is what Nancy advises, which is a slow and steady approach. Mind you, this doesn't mean we're advocating counting all these calories. That's the last, last resort, because, as I pointed out in chapter 5, the math of caloric deficits involves so much guesswork that you might as well not even bother. Nancy's assertion is simply to let you know starvation is not good. It won't help you achieve your goals.

The One Time It's Okay to Be Hungry

The one time it's okay to be hungry is before bed. This sounds simple, but it's actually a powerful weight loss tool that can stop you from ingesting a few hundred unnecessary calories.

Remember what France Bellisle wrote about the obese eating little early in the day and then getting night-eating syndrome? The idea is to stay fueled during the day so you *don't* overeat at night. If you can go to bed a little hungry, tomorrow morning is a new day when you start fresh. Unless you go to bed so hungry that you wake up in the middle of the night needing to eat. That's too hungry.

For the rest of the day, there's an old adage that says, "Eat until you are eight-tenths full." It's good advice. Focus on being *satisfied* throughout the day, not full or *stuffed*. Stuffed is for Thanksgiving and Christmas.

For emotional eaters who have trouble with stopping at satisfied, try portioning out the appropriate amount of food in advance, and once it's finished, remove yourself from any additional food temptations whenever possible. If you're feeling stressed and overly tempted, taking a walk is always a good choice. If you'll be walking past places that serve food, don't bring money.

Tips for Going to Bed a Little Hungry

You may find, a few hours after dinner, that you still want to eat. Here are some tips to prevent that:

- Realize that you've been busy all day and now have a chance to relax. This may be boredom you're feeling instead of hunger. You want to do something, and eating is doing something, so you eat. Well, don't eat. Do something else. Like stretch. Keep a yoga mat handy and reach for that instead of food.

- Take a shower. Its rewarding effects can feel just as good as food.
- Brush your teeth. Can't eat again after you've brushed your teeth, right?
- Drink some hot herbal tea. Make it hot enough that it takes time to drink. Don't burn your tongue or your crotch, though.
- Clean a toilet. Seriously, who can eat after doing that?
- Go to bed and read.
- Go to bed and do . . . other stuff. If you're having a tough time talking your partner into this, tell him or her that it's part of your weight loss strategy. Who knows? It could work.

KEEPING IT SIMPLE: OUR ONE-LINE DIET PLAN

I often wonder how people come up with their hyper-convoluted diet plans based on . . . God knows what. Was the guy who wrote about choosing foods based on your blood type suffering from a rectal-cranial inversion? Did he have a look around up there, then pull that diet out of his ass?

Dr. David Katz told me the challenge with truth is that it is not a one-liner. Behold our one-liner!

Gradually replace bad stuff with good stuff.

Sorry, David. I guess there is more to it than that. Again, behold!

Our Three-point Mission Statement

We have three points we'd like you to memorize. Taken together, they will help you follow that one-liner, and that one-liner will help you lose weight. The first two points were originally spoken by Jack LaLanne.

1. *"If it tastes good, spit it out."* I need to clarify this one. Swap the word *good* for *amazing*. Fruit and steak and lots of other things taste good, even great, but chocolate and cheesecake and popcorn chicken and

maple fudge taste amazing. If your taste buds are being manipulated to the point that you can't control consumption, that qualifies as "amazing." Also, you don't have to spit out the amazing all the time. Instead, just remember to limit such things to the occasional indulgence. This is about a *reduction* in highly palatable food, not complete elimination.

2. *"If man made it, don't eat it."* That's pretty clear, but there are exceptions. There are whole-wheat whole-grain bread products that are awesome. There is good oatmeal you can buy. If things are close to being in a natural state yet are still "processed," that can be okay. It's the highly refined stuff you need to watch out for. There are a number of resources free from the Food and Drug Administration that can make you more literate when it comes to reading labels. To find all these resources, google this phrase: "FDA Nutrition Facts Label Programs and Materials." (A google-worthy phrase for Canucks is "Health Canada Nutrition Labelling.") Overall, you want to focus on foods with few ingredients listed. As my wife tells her patients, "If nature made it that way, go big." Sticking to the outside aisle of the grocery store can help with this, because this is where the fresher, single-ingredient foods such as dairy, produce and meat are found.

3. *"Put better fuel in the tank."* Let's think back to chapter 4 and give credit where it's due on this one: to Dr. Katz (I have a man-crush on this guy). When we exercise, we're more likely to focus on putting better fuel in the tank, and this in turn provides the psychological boost we need to help us get over the "because I exercised" reward mentality that Dr. Freedhoff mentioned. You want to perform better, and that requires rocket-fuel go juice. When you're about to eat something, ask yourself this question: "Is this rocket-fuel go juice?" If it's not, you know what to do.

All this amounts to mindful, not mindless, eating. You need to *pay attention to your food*, not just reach for something and start shoveling it in. Paying attention to what you're eating is perhaps the most powerful tool we have at our disposal to reduce caloric intake.[9]

Incrementally Decreasing the Reward Value of Food

This is the basis of our "one-liner" diet plan. The "bad stuff" has a high reward value; you need to replace this with "good stuff" that has a lower reward value.

Let's throw around some guestimated numbers here. Looking at North American waistlines, I think it's not too far off to say about 80 percent of calories ingested by overweight people are "high-reward" calories (ones that have a high hedonic value, i.e., they taste amazing). Maybe we're off, but for the sake of argument let's just say we're correct on that number so we can give you an idea of an incremental program of cutting back on the reward value of food.

The food reward hypothesis of obesity states that eating higher-flavor foods leads to higher levels of body fat. There is enough research supporting this concept to choke a sarlacc—the nasty pit-of-death monster that Jabba the Hutt wanted to throw Han Solo into. (Note to self: when you have to explain your jokes, they are no longer funny.) Anyway, check out this mega endnote.[10] It's kind of a "well, duh" thing. If you focus on eating food that tastes delicious, you will eat more of it. The double whammy is that this food packs in more calories. Focusing on a diet of super-yummy food = you gaining weight.

"If it tastes really, really good, you probably shouldn't eat it," actor Michael Biehn told me. Biehn, who has been known for his lean and mean physique (which comes in handy when battling terminators and aliens), said, "I just think it's common sense that if something tastes great like a potato chip or a French fry or a Big Mac, that it's not going to be good for you. But if you eat a piece of broccoli, you can just tell it's a good choice." Yup. We know, but we don't always do.

If you're a typical North American wanting to lose weight, eating 80 percent of your calories as high-reward calories, you're eating these for pleasure-based, hedonically motivated reasons. This also means only 20 percent of calories are consumed for homeostatic, fueling-based reasons.

In order to successfully lose weight, you need to change this. In fact, you need to almost transpose those two numbers, from an 80 percent pleasure / 20 percent fuel split to the other way around. So how do you do this? *Gradually.*

- *First level of dietary change:* Ratio shifts to 60 percent of calories pleasure-focused / 40 percent fuel.
- *Second level of dietary change:* Ratio shifts to 40 percent of calories pleasure-focused / 60 percent fuel.
- *Third level of dietary change:* Ratio shifts to 20 percent of calories pleasure-focused / 80 percent fuel.

And I want you to meticulously measure that down to the last calorie.

Please tell me you didn't believe that last sentence. You know me better than that by now.

These three levels are *approximations* of what you're about to go through in Stage III. In case we haven't made it clear, it's the highly refined, amazing-tasting food that makes people fat. You've got to cut that down and replace it with healthier, higher- performance real food that still tastes good but not mouthgasm good.

Dammit, I promised I wasn't going to use that word anymore. My bad.

The Critical Component: Adopting the *Replacement* Mentality

Professor Richard Mattes and I talked about the assumption that eating large quantities of fruits and vegetables reduces calorie intake later in the day. This is the "crowding out" hypothesis that's popular among some holistic nutritionists because it's hippie granola thinking that *telling people to cut bad stuff will, like, harsh up their vibe, man.* They think fruits and vegetables have some miraculous power to make you stop eating bad foods. Well, they don't.

"We did a study making people eat five fruits and vegetables a day and they *gained weight* because they didn't change the rest of their diet," Mattes told me. "It doesn't work from a crowding-out perspective. It doesn't magically cause you to eat less. You must make a conscious decision to replace one food with another."

In coming chapters we *will* harsh up your vibe by getting you to cut junk, and we'll offer a better replacement. The replacements will not taste as good, but they will be lower in calories, more satiating and healthier and they will fuel physical performance. You will be eating food that, as Dr. Katz says, loves you back.

We've brainstormed to make the food replacement process as painless as possible, both from a neurological standpoint and from a practical / time management / lifestyle perspective. We've selected "stop eating this / start eating this" rules based on what will be easiest for you to handle as well as lead to a positive outcome.

And know that these dietary changes become easier with time. Part of it is craving related, but another part is just practice. You get practiced at making the right choices and knowing what's good and what's bad. You build skill power.

Think of the last time you started a new job. You sucked at first. You didn't know where anything was, how to navigate the bureaucracy, how deep the water was or how many sharks were swimming in it. Anyway, you sucked. But with time and practice you got better. You got efficient. You gained confidence and skill. Diet and exercise are no different.

On the craving side, a 2007 article in *Appetite* interviewed 284 people and determined that after spending time on a reduced fat diet, subjects had a declining preference for fatty foods.[11] It takes time, but junk food will lose its hold.

The Challenge of Keeping Track

Yes, Virginia, it's all about the calories.

It's not that you have to count them, but you *must be aware* of what you're eating. If you follow the replacement rules we lay out in Stage III, it's an almost guaranteed way to lose weight. Almost. You can still blow it if you mindlessly eat without realizing you've done so. It's a common trait among heavier people to underestimate by a wide margin how many calories they consume in a day.[12]

Counting calories is a last resort, but *calorie awareness* can be a valuable tool. Get used to understanding how many calories are in everything you eat. In *The End of Overeating*, Dr. David Kessler promoted counter-conditioning, a psychological technique to develop negative associations with the food you love in order to decrease your longing for it. He said highly palatable food needs to go from being a friend to "a detested enemy."[13]

That's going overboard. Such thinking gives junk food power over you by making it appealing as forbidden fruit. Instead, try viewing junk food as a number—a number of calories. At the grocery store, look at that blueberry pie. Read the label and see how many calories are in it. It may say how many for one-eighth of the pie, but realize you'll probably eat one-quarter and do the math. Understand how many calories that is. Think about how satisfying it is or is *not* going to be. Determine if it's worth it.

Over time, you can figure out how many calories are in many things. You can measure potato chips, chocolate, ice cream, pizza slices, burgers and fries; smartphones can give you caloric content on the fly. Each time you're tempted, view the desired treat as a number of calories, and make an informed decision about whether the reward merits the caloric cost.

If you find you're still not successful, a food journal in which you write everything down can be beneficial.

Eat Well Because You Exercised

I want you to remember all you've learned thus far about how highly palatable food, food cues and the food industry at large manipulate you. We want you to begin to see junk food less as a source of constant pleasure, comfort and need and more with wariness, caution and an eye toward the occasional indulgence.

Don't hate the junk food. Instead, work toward reaching a place where it doesn't hold so much power over you, where you eat only the best and favorite ones on occasion to treat yourself.

When you begin making dietary changes, remember that you are powerful. Exercise is making you this way. It's helping to make you strong not just physically but mentally. It's giving you the power to make wise food choices. And, when necessary, it's giving you the power to resist making bad choices.

Remember when Dr. Freedhoff said that "because I exercised" are the three dangerous words that cripple weight management? It's time to turn that reward mentality around. Look at healthy food choices and say to yourself, "I can learn to like this. I can make most of my food choices good ones. I can resist eating junk food. I can do this."

Because I exercised.

7

GET MOTIVATED: GOAL SETTING AND THE SCIENCE OF BEHAVIOR CHANGE

I was taught that the way of progress was neither swift nor easy.

—MARIE CURIE

An important part of the preparation process is complete—we blew away the myths of diet and exercise and how they affect weight loss—but there is still more preparation to be done before you get ready to "Do." In order to become a person who can follow through, you must first be motivated to change.

My friend Dr. Peter Sargious is a specialist in internal medicine, with a research interest in chronic disease prevention and management. He has learned the importance of making time to exercise and eat healthily, and he told me of the consequences for those who don't.

"In my years of clinical practice and in my field of research I see the implications of not prioritizing health among the other demands people face in their lives," he said. "Unfortunately, I sometimes see the final outcome of these patients' choices later on in the hospital, dealing with chronic disease."

Sargious also explained that you can't be as good a parent, spouse or employee if your health is suffering. "If people imagine these demands necessitate that they place a lower priority on their health, they may discover their lack of attention has a bigger negative effect on fulfilling these duties. Over the short term it may seem logical, but in the long term it's self-defeating."

With Sargious's words in mind, and while we're still in this "preparing" stage, I want to remind you of some words I used to close the introduction of this book. Losing it right is about changing who you are. It is not a list of actions but rather someone you become.

Sticking to a regimen of exercise and healthy eating is not easy. Just having a list of dos and don'ts will not make the tough decisions of reprioritizing your life magically happen. It's a process of integration. Remember, don't just do this; be this.

BEFORE YOU START

In the introduction, I mentioned that adherence to this plan—or any other plan, for that matter—won't transform you into a bikini model in a month. Age, illness, genetics or your life situation may put you at a disadvantage. Given all that, you should set goals that are achievable (we will show you how).

This doesn't, however, mean you shouldn't be ambitious. The slow road can take you a long way. This journey to a healthier you is about incremental improvements, which involve revisiting your goals regularly and making adaptations based on what you've learned and the new person you are becoming. Here are a few things to keep in mind before you start.

Avoid the Toxic Mind-set

Forget that stuff about "only minutes a day." That word "only" implies that exercise is a form of punishment to be endured in order to achieve a specific end. The people who use that phrase, or phrases like it, are saying, "We know you hate this, so we've come up with a *miracle* method that minimizes the time spent doing something you detest."

It's a crock, not to mention a toxic mind-set. Exercise is *not* punishment. It's an awesome and righteous lifestyle to be embraced with passion and vigor until the end of your days.

I feel as if I'm freaking you out. If the old me read the above two paragraphs, he'd be rolling his eyes. Don't worry; we'll get you there.

Screw the Scale

When it comes to getting in shape, most people focus on reducing the numbers on the scale as their primary goal. I don't advocate this.

Trust me: I know how powerful the words "weight loss" are. Any time I write an online article with the words "weight loss," "belly fat" or "metabolism" in the title, the clicks go through the roof.

But here I am, in all seriousness, telling you that you may want to consider burying your scale in the storage room.

The scale is not always your friend. It lies. It is not a measure of your health or fitness, and it doesn't account for muscle gained. It does not in any way represent your worth as a human being.

There are, however, numbers worth tracking as you go on this journey, such as miles run, walked or cycled. Laps swum or weight lifted. Classes attended and hills climbed. Fruits and vegetables consumed and healthy meals prepared. Those are good numbers to track. Those are *motivating* numbers.

Other ways to track progress, or tell if you're backsliding, are how pants feel, which belt notch you use, how much belly you can grab and how you look in the mirror. Such things can provide more accurate information than a scale.

Yes, there are a number of studies showing that daily weighing helps with weight loss, but I'm suggesting that tracking those other numbers and milestones is an even more powerful motivator. This approach is more Zen-like, the numbers move faster, and it represents gaining instead of losing. You gain strength, speed, stamina and overall physical butt-kickery. Recall the brain-boosting effects of exercise that we learned about in chapter 4; I'll bet if you took before and after IQ tests, you'd see a jump in those results too.

The visual aspect—that "how you look in the mirror" thing—can be the best motivator of all. Simply seeing how much better you look gives much more powerful reinforcement than a number on a machine. Think how cool it will be when your friends say, "Have you lost weight?" and you can reply with honesty, "I don't know."

(When they ask your secret, please tell them it's this book.)

Years ago, I was director of marketing for the Faculty of Kinesiology at the University of Calgary. We picked two overweight students, Audrey and Rory, to go through a five-month fitness challenge. The before and after photos were astounding. Both made tremendous transformations not just in their looks but in their athleticism and health as well.

Guess what the scale said? Audrey lost a *whopping* six pounds. And Rory? He *gained* a pound. That's the difference muscle can make. As I said, the scale lies.

Your body weight is going to be what it's going to be. Obsessively tracking it doesn't help you feel the love. Yes, if you follow the advice in this book you most likely will lose weight, perhaps a lot. But try to see that as a side benefit rather than an overarching motivator. The main goal is a happier, healthier you.

If you can do the scale in a way that doesn't depress you, knowing that weight loss will be slow, then feel free to use it. I'm not saying you can't. But if you want to transcend it, if you want to bury that sucker under a pile of old tax returns in the basement, you go.

I will continue to mention weight loss in this book because many of the regular people I interviewed as I was writing have lost considerable amounts. I include it because it gives you an idea of what they accomplished. I'm not saying you should never weigh yourself again; I am saying don't let the scale rule your life. Focus on improving the good numbers I mentioned above, and just let your weight be what it will be. You'll wind up healthier and happier.

Being motivated to change doesn't require that you hate who you are right now. Seeing yourself with shame is not a healthy starting point. Yes, people who lose a lot of weight and get in good shape are to be admired, but this does not mean those who are overweight should be shunned.

Even if you're only aiming to lose 10 pounds, don't look at the extra fat on your butt, thighs or belly with disgust. As mentioned in chapter 3, this is not a healthy attitude, so reject the stigma. Embrace the new body you achieve and strive to improve it further, but don't hate the old one. Love your body and do nice things for it.

It's the only one you'll ever have.

SETTING GOALS

Okay. Now that we've got that out of the way, we can get down to the business of setting goals, because as Lewis Carroll said, "If you don't know where you're going, any road will get you there." Besides, having at least part of one eye on the prize will keep you motivated, but it's important to understand there are different types of goals.

You know how, if you're watching World Cup soccer (football—whatever) and someone scores, the announcer yells, *"GOOOOOOOOO OAAAAAAAAAALLLLLL!!!!!"*?

Yeah, me neither. I personally don't spend much time watching sports. I prefer to engage in them instead.

Back on topic: Scoring a goal in a big match is an exciting, visible, definable outcome. But what most people don't see when they tune in to the game is the process involved in this achievement, the years and years of intensive effort that make the outcome goal a reality.

So let's break it down and figure out how achieving goals really works.

SMART Goals

A 1985 article in the *Journal of Sport Psychology* notes that the type of goal you set can make a difference to your outcome. Goals that are more specific and difficult can lead to a better performance than vague or easy ones.[1] I'm a fan of aiming high. That way, if you only make it 80 percent of the way, you're still thrilled with the outcome.

"The evidence is very strong that people who set SMART goals are more likely to pursue those goals," says sport psychologist Jim Taylor. SMART goals are

- Specific
- Measurable
- Actionable
- Realistic
- Timely

Putting a picture of a fitness model on the fridge and saying, "I want to look like that" is not a SMART goal. Saying, "I intend to lose 20 pounds of fat and gain 10 pounds of muscle in the next six months" is.

Your goals need to be realistic, and unfortunately realism is a little hard to come by in a world where there is such a *huge* amount of bovine droppings in the popular media promising that you can lose [*insert ridiculously high number here*] pounds of fat in only [*insert stupidly short period of time here*].

The fact is, getting in shape is hard. And slow. And hard. If it were as easy as those Internet pop-up ads promise, everyone would look like Brangelina from the neck down. If you need a dose of reality, shop at Walmart.

Aim high, sure, but stay within the realm of the possible. Figure out not only what is physiologically feasible for your age, gender, genetics and health status but *psychologically* achievable. The older, heavier and more time constrained you are, the more challenging it is to achieve ambitious goals. If you're younger, not too overweight and have fewer demands on your time, the term "the sky is the limit" becomes far more applicable. There is no scientific formula to determine precisely what you can or cannot achieve (and sustain). I've seen some amazing transformations in my day. Everyone is unique, and figuring out what is possible for *you* is part of the process you'll go through in Stage III.

If you have lofty goals, understand that it's going to take some serious mental toughness and consistent effort to achieve them. Then you'll have to sustain that effort to keep your new shape. You can't go back to old habits and keep the new you.

Now that we've clarified how goal setting works, it's time to actually do it. This is an important part of the preparation process. For this lifestyle overhaul thing to really work, you'll need two types of goals—outcome goals and process goals. Let's start with outcome.

Outcome Goals

Outcome goals help you sort out where you want to end up. They can also be referred to as your long-term goals. Outcome goals—which should be SMART goals, remember—can be motivated by whatever it takes to get and keep you committed. Here are some examples behind most outcome goals:

- VANITY: Things like the weight or inches lost and muscle gained mentioned above. If you want, you can also have a realistic magazine photo of what you want to look like, or a photo of yourself from years past, in the shape that you want to recapture. I put vanity first on this list because I know what a powerful motivator it is.
- HEALTH: Lowered cholesterol and blood pressure, reduced cancer / Alzheimer's / cardiac risk, amelioration of debilitating conditions.
- PERFORMANCE: Finishing a race (or perhaps setting an ambitious time in which to finish it); being able to do an intense fitness class start to finish; being able to lift a certain amount of weight; being able to take the stairs at work without stopping to rest or feeling as if you're going to cough up a kidney.

Most of the fittest people I know are equally motivated by vanity, health and performance. I like the idea of focusing outcome goals on one-third vanity, one-third health and one-third performance, but it's important to make these mutually inclusive. Stimulants and extreme dieting can help achieve a vanity goal, but will sacrifice health and even physical performance. Since using vanity as a motivator has potential risks, it's worth further investigation.

Embracing (a Little) Vanity
You're so vain, you probably think this section is about you.

Carly Simon may be down on vanity, but I'm cool with it, as long as you don't go off the deep end and pull a Heidi Montag, wandering into the plastic surgeon's office and ordering the Barbie Doll–*Muppet Show* special.

"People are hardwired to strive to look better because it brings benefits throughout life, be it in mate selection, employment opportunities, salary or life in general," I was told by Gordon Patzer, a professor of business administration at Roosevelt University in Chicago and the author of six books on the physical attractiveness phenomenon.

"While many people state they are pursuing fitness for health reasons, the truth is that these are often secondary to their desire to look better," he said.

But vanity can go sideways if we put too much emphasis on it. "It can cross a line where we get into anorexia and bulimia," Patzer said, "or people who do too much exercise and cause injury. We can also go too far by getting radical plastic surgery, taking anabolic steroids or dangerous weight loss supplements, or going on crash diets."

"After my second child I felt like I had lost my attractiveness," Susan Sadler, a 40-year-old mother of two in Alberta, told me. "I knew that if I got in shape, I would look better and feel better. I started seeing results, and that was a big motivator." It must be, because between running and weightlifting, Susan exercises hard six hours a week now.

Stefan Pinto now lives in Los Angeles, but it was his Wall Street job that made him fat. "I saw a photo with my stomach sticking out, and I couldn't believe how much weight I had put on," he said.

Transformation was a slow process, but it brought amazing results and being discovered by a modeling scout. "Making visible progress for me was what made the act of exercise more enjoyable," Stefan said. (If you want to see just how much progress he made, google him.)

Vanity motivates me as well. My website is called "Body for Wife," and I do like looking good for her. There's a healthy way you can use vanity as motivation to eat well and exercise. It's not shallow if it helps you live a healthier lifestyle. When I decided to make abdominal definition a goal, I went about achieving it in a smart and healthy way: I cut my beer intake in half and junk food by around two-thirds, and I ran more. Conversely, rocker Iggy Pop got his six-pack abs via heroin and sex with a stream of groupies. Some may disagree, but I think my way is better.

Believe it or not, so does Paul Stanley. Those who know the band KISS know lead singer Paul Stanley's "Starchild" costume reveals much of his torso. At 60 years old, he fought to stay lean for the band's 2013 "Monster" tour.

"Nobody wants to see a fat guy in tights," Stanley told me. "That wouldn't be fair to the fans."

Although he has a desire to look good onstage, he keeps health paramount. "I think vanity in some degree is a great incentive," Stanley said. "Narcissism can be a problem, but taking pride in yourself, you shouldn't see that as detrimental. We should try to look our best, because the road to looking our best is one that involves being healthy. When I look my best, more than likely I'm also feeling my best."

Get an idea of what you want to achieve long term. Figure out what your outcome is. Perhaps write it down and stick it somewhere you can see it. Again, aim high, so that if you only make it 80 percent of the way there, you're still thrilled. Also, if you achieve your outcome goals, set new and more ambitious ones. I've been working out since 1993, and just two years ago I thought the idea of completing an Ironman triathlon was crazy, but now I'm totally planning to do it. Always having something to reach for makes sustainability of health and weight loss a lot easier.

Now let's look at how you achieve those goals.

Process Goals—Exercise

To achieve the outcome, you must focus on the process.

Losing weight, building muscle, lowering cardiac risk factors, improving physical performance, etcetera, all require effort. You need to do things such as exercise and eat healthily (and restrict calories) to accomplish your outcome goals; these processes can all be broken down.

You do *not* just jump into being a hard-core workout warrior overnight. You will hate it and you *will* hurt yourself. So don't.

Instead, remember to be the tortoise and not the hare. Start off with a week of exercise that's only a little out of your comfort zone, but commit to push your efforts in increments until you achieve your own personal level of "good enough."

You need to push these increments along the following lines:

- the frequency with which you exercise
- the intensity at which you exercise
- the length of time spent exercising
- the difficulty level of the types of exercises you engage in

Now, I don't know you or your capabilities, so I'm going to offer a pretty easy scenario as an example here. You can push harder than this, as long as you don't end up hating the process.

Learn to Crawl

"I told my husband, who is 64 and retired, that he had to help me be motivated, and we just started walking together," said Charlene Casey, a 51-year-old records manager in Los Angeles.

Casey had never been an exerciser and had become obese. And so she and her husband started off easily, just a couple of miles of walking each time. But with each passing month they went farther and farther, to the point that within a few months they found they were walking six miles each outing, three times a week. What's more, Casey got some inexpensive dumbbells, exercise bands, medicine balls and an inflatable fitness ball, and set up a simple home gym. For instruction, she found videos on YouTube. And then the exercise became a gateway behavior to better eating.

"I lost 70 pounds in six months," she said. And she's maintaining. Oh, and her husband lost over 30 pounds. And this inspired their adult daughter to exercise and eat better, and she lost over 50 pounds. Slow and steady can get you there. Believe it.

Create a Routine

In the first week of your lifestyle overhaul you might do something easy and short, say just a couple of 30-minute aquacize classes. Now, aquacize doesn't burn many calories or do much for improving physical performance, but doing something easy like this is a critical first step: it creates a routine of regular exercise. Don't expect to lose a single pound of fat during these initial stages, but do celebrate your accomplishment of regular exercise. If you do something physical twice a week—even walking—you're doing better than most of the modern world, so give yourself a pat on the back.

Really, if you go from doing nothing to doing something physical—anything—a couple of times a week, this is a *major accomplishment* and an important first step. Be proud of yourself. Just don't use it as an excuse for chocolate cheesecake. It doesn't work that way.

Push a Little Harder

When what was uncomfortable becomes comfortable, when you have the routine of a small amount of regular physical activity ingrained in your lifestyle, get a little uncomfortable again. Don't stick with just aquacize—move on to something harder.

Say it takes six weeks before you're starting to feel as if this class is easy. In Week Seven, kick it up a notch. Keep the class going, but add a 30-minute power walk.

In Week 10, maybe you'll decide aquacize is too easy and trade it in for Spinning or Zumba classes or something else. Also, you decide to power-walk twice a week.

In Week 15 those power walks are turning into jogs.

In Week 20 you decide to hire a personal trainer to check out weight-lifting and start adding two 45-minute training sessions a week.

In Week 25 those jogs have become runs and you've registered for a 5K race. Maybe even a 10K.

And one day, you do a half marathon and then maybe a marathon, and so on.

Get the idea?

"It takes a while to get good at a sport," Olympic champion kayaker Adam Van Koeverden told me. "To be good at anything just requires a ton of practice. I've paddled a kayak over 80,000 kilometers in my life, and that's why I'm good at it."

He's an Olympian, which means he's an outlier, but know that gaining competence in any activity is going to take time. Lifting weights is more complex than lifting heavy things up and putting them back down again. Running takes time to master. Not everyone is a born swimmer. Yoga takes . . . I don't have a clue what it takes to get good at yoga. A lot of classes, I'll bet.

It's what you do in the short term that makes the difference long term. Focus on the process, and the outcome takes care of itself.

Follow Through

One way to make sure you both create and follow through on your process goals is to take your chosen physical activities and create a monthly calendar of what you're going to do and stick it on the fridge. Then I want you to relish trying your best to tick off every single one of those scheduled exercise sessions as "Done."

The reason I want you to do this is that "when, where and how" details boost adherence.

"When you have a strong commitment to a desired outcome [i.e., a goal] this has some effect on the rate of goal attainment," Peter Gollwitzer, a professor of psychology at New York University, told me. "But when in addition you spell out the 'when, where and how' of goal striving in terms of *if-then* plans, you get a much stronger rate of goal attainment. It's about twice as high." (More on "if-then" plans later in this chapter.)

And it's not the quantity of detail you spell out in your plans, Gollwitzer says, but the quality of it. It needs to cover how you want to deal with your personal obstacles to achieving your goals. But this doesn't mean you jump right into fitness like an apocalyptic lemming. Slow and steady is what wins this race.

Who knows, maybe seeing your workout schedule on the fridge will help you make wiser eating decisions when you open that fridge door as well.

At the end of the month, evaluate, make adaptations and come up with a more ambitious schedule. Repeat again and again, until this becomes second nature and you feel that you don't need the schedule anymore.

Process Goals—Eating

Remember that a good and realistic lifestyle overhaul plan has two equal parts: exercise and eating. If you set only exercise-related process goals, you'll be ignoring a vital component, and your results will suffer. You need to take the same process goal approach with eating as you do with exercise. Luckily, the method is the same: slow and steady.

And don't get all hung up on doing this right away—for one simple, soul-crushing reason: the diet part is often harder than exercise, so we want you to wait. Sucks, I know, but it's true. Here's why:

- Adopting exercise is taking on a good habit, and it's easier to start something good than it is to quit something bad, like overeating junk.
- Highly palatable food, as you saw in chapter 2, has addictive properties. With junk food you're working to break a compulsion.
- Remember chapter 1? Junk food is everywhere. It will take a buildup of mental resources via exercise to learn to control yourself around it.
- For exercise, you need to be motivated only for the time you are exercising. I consider myself a hard-core exerciser. I average eight to 10 hours a week, at either moderate or high intensity. That leaves 158 or so hours in the rest of the week when I don't need to be motivated to work out. Conversely, diet is 24/7. You can be good on your diet for days and then undo it all in an hour of crazed gluttony.

So, if you find dietary changes as daunting as most people do, wait for a bit. Get the exercise thing down first. Focus all your initial energies on this, build up your health-specific willpower and FORGET ABOUT LOSING WEIGHT FOR NOW! It's critical to remember that in the majority of cases, exercise INDIRECTLY causes weight loss by strengthening mental capabilities to focus on healthier, calorie-restricted eating. The number of calories it burns for most people makes only a small contribution to the caloric deficits necessary to lose weight. I'll say it again: lean bodies are made in the kitchen.

Exercise will make you stronger and faster and blah, blah, blah—I already told you all this. It will provide you with your "replacement addiction" as well, inhibit your desire for junk food and other things that are bad for you, and smarten up your brain so you're better at following through on a plan. It's also going to make you start *feeling* like a healthy person, and when that happens you'll want to start *eating* like a healthy person.

So know that the dietary changes have to come, and start making those changes when you're ready.

Week after week you can add in healthier foods while also removing the garbage ones. It's important to remember that healthy food is a replacement, not an addition. As we've mentioned, unconsciously "crowding out" junk food with healthy choices doesn't happen. It needs to be a conscious decision.

If you eat only one serving of fruit a day, try for two in Week One. But you need to eat this fruit *instead of* eating something lousy. Also, if you eat out 10 times a week, Week One could see you cut back to nine times, and so on. You get the idea. Incremental improvements can lead to your desired outcomes.

The Long Road to Success

"A journey of a thousand miles begins with a single step," said some wise dude from long ago.

Fine, it was Chinese philosopher Lao-tzu in the sixth century BCE. Google rocks.

Psychologists have observed that it doesn't matter if it's one person planning an individual goal, such as getting in shape, or a large team planning to build a railway or the Chunnel; people will consistently underestimate the time, energy and resources it takes to accomplish goals.[2] So be patient.

Take your first step, then your second, then a third, and eventually you will travel your thousand miles. Then you can keep right on traveling.

THE SCIENCE OF MOTIVATION

In case you hadn't noticed, Margaret and I are kind of into the science thing. We like rational theories substantiated via facts. We dig the scientific method.

Let's put that on hold for a bit. With life-changing events, sometimes you just have to feel it.

I want you to imagine someone who loves to exercise. I want you to imagine this person is you. You went from someone who hated it to someone who finds such great pleasure in physical activity that it comes to define you as a person. I want you to imagine this changing your life so that, years from now, people think of you as a workout warrior.

This is going to be hard. In fact, it may be one of the hardest things you ever do. But you can power through. You can learn to feel the love. You can make exercise and healthy eating a part of who you are.

The Ordinary Miracle

Still waiting for that weight loss miracle? They do happen, but it's not going to come via something that magically melts fat; it's more like a spiritual awakening.

Jen Hamel is a mother of two small children in Edmonton. Six years ago she was a smoker, a daily Slurpee drinker and a fast food eater. She was sedentary, unhappy and weighed 205 pounds.

"There was a catalyst," she told me. "I saw a group photo from a family reunion and finally realized what was happening to me. The next day I saw commercials for Turbo Jam fitness DVDs, and because my kids were babies it made sense to exercise at home."

Jen bought a DVD. And that led to many more changes in her life.

"It started with exercise, and then I began making small changes in my diet," she said. "It took me a year to lose 65 pounds." But it didn't stop there. "Gradually, over time, I just became a fitness freak." She's down to 135 pounds, runs in Spartan races, does half marathons and competes in a women's strength and fitness challenge called Femsport.

New Jen's lifestyle became the polar opposite of Old Jen's lifestyle. She was in the death spiral, and she got into the Virtuous Cycle. And she's still in it, working as a personal trainer with an eye on her first marathon.

What happened to Jen isn't an image-of-the-Virgin-Mary-in-a-grilled-cheese-sandwich miracle, but it's a miracle nonetheless. People *can* change for the better. Have no faith in the false promises of charlatans and snake oil salesmen. Have faith in yourself.

It happened to Jen. It's happened to countless others. It can happen to you.

Embracing Exercise Is Not Easy

I know you have doubts.

Most people don't exercise, and they don't want to start. It's harder to move than to not move. There is no time. It's painful. It makes you smelly. You don't know what to do. People might make fun of you. You can get hurt. It costs money. None of your friends do it. Your TiVo is full of stuff to watch. There are Internet friends who require your attention.

The exercise lifestyle is not an easy one to embrace. Many try and fail. Granted, I believe the reason they fail is that they approach it with the wrong attitude, improper motivations and a lack of quality information. In other words, they've been listening to the bs spewed by Weight Loss Inc.

As we've shown, falling in love with exercise is something that *happens*. There is no "Secret" to "Law of Attraction" the flab away. No one ever had a pair of calorie-burning underpants change their life. How many owe fit and healthy bodies to a supplement or an ab-toning contraption from an infomercial?

But going from couch potato to workout warrior—and having it change your life—is something that happens every day. There are people who are overweight, inactive and with unhealthy diets who will start exercising, and they will learn not to hate it, then like it and eventually . . . love it. And then that will change everything else, including the way they eat. Remember all that stuff from chapter 3 about the benefits of exercise and healthy eating? It opens the door to a better life.

One more time. It happens. It can happen to you.

Every day, someone falls in love with his or her soul mate. Every day, someone stands up to a bully. Every day, someone risks her or his life to save another. Every day, a mother makes a child's awful day all better with just a hug. Every day, someone does the right thing even when the wrong thing was so much easier. Every day, ordinary things happen that appear miraculous. I don't believe in weight loss miracles, but real-life miracles happen all the time.

Maybe this is the turning point. Maybe this is the end of the yoyo. Maybe the epiphany is on the edge of your consciousness, yearning to burst through.

Maybe you're due for your real-life miracle.

Okay, I apologize for getting over the top with all that cheese. It's time to science this sucker up again. And by science, I'm not talking about Tony Robbins neuro-cognitive-linguistic-association-programming horse pucky. There are proven theories to back up this power of positive thinking. One of them is called . . .

The Theory of Planned Behavior (TPB)

This influential theory was formulated by Icek Ajzen in 1985. Since then, it has been studied and applied by numerous researchers,[3] many of whom found it to be a good predictor of who will adopt a new behavior and who won't.[4] So what? Well, if the research says people who think and believe a certain way are more likely to be successful in adopting new behaviors such as diet and exercise, maybe you should try to change your thinking and beliefs to something along those lines. It's just a thought.

Ajzen's model focuses a lot on intention, stating that most human behavior is goal oriented. Intention is generated by two things: does the subject have a positive or a negative attitude about the behavior, and does the subject believe others close to him or her support this change in behavior.[5]

So here's the "well, duh" moment: if you have a positive attitude about a new behavior and you believe others think you should engage in this new behavior, it increases your *intention* of engaging in that behavior. It ain't rocket surgery.

Next step? Add to your level of intention your "perceived behavioral control," which is how much control you think you have over your life. Do you believe you can make the necessary rearrangements to your schedule to fit in exercise?[6] If you answered no to that question, you need to go back and reread chapter 1 about work-life balance.

TPB is a predictive model. If you score high on all three questions, you're more likely to engage in the new behavior. This is why it's important to train your brain. Incidentally, having a positive attitude and believing you have control over your behaviors have been shown to be the two most important factors, whereas the influence of what you believe others think is less important.[7] So if others around you are naysayers, screw those guys.

The "Theory" of Planned Competition

A great way to engage TPB is to register for a race or other competition, because doing so shows you have that "positive attitude" about your ability to follow through. For example, I know a number of people who have kick-started diet and exercise by registering for races and physique competitions.

A profound example is Wes Daniel's story.

Daniel, a property manager who lives in California, lost his partner to HIV/AIDS and cancer in 2004, and Daniel's doctor told him he was dying too—from obesity. "At 40 years old and 275 pounds, I was on a path to an early death," Daniel said. "My doctor kept telling me to change my lifestyle, and I had tried different exercises and diet plans, but nothing stuck."

Then Daniel found his exercise passion. "I had heard so many good things about the AIDS LifeCycle experience," he said. "I started training and lost 65 pounds." A healthier diet played a role, but the ride was the impetus to change.

The AIDS LifeCycle event is a seven-day, 545-mile bike ride from San Francisco to Los Angeles. When I spoke to Daniel, he was about to do the ride for a second time. Having that long ride on his "to do" list forces him to keep his fitness up during the year.

Another key aspect of a positive attitude is feeling confident and competent in what you're about to do; it's called . . .

Self-efficacy Theory

Say you walk past a gym and see a Nike sign proclaiming, Just Do It! You walk in, succumb to the high-pressure sales pitch and buy a membership. Then you attempt a workout using your *Magnum P.I.* shorts from high school with no clue what you're doing or how to use the equipment. Perhaps you hurt yourself. Also, you find the place is full of arrogant muscle heads with snake and skull tattoos running from knuckles to neck. You hate it and never go back.

That was a bad investment. Putting the self-efficacy theory into practice would have helped prevent this, because it's all about taking the time to learn about a new behavior and gradually develop confidence to ensure a more positive experience. Although it's not as catchy as Nike's slogan, self-efficacy is central to our program of Learn, Prepare, Do. Developed by Albert Bandura, a Stanford University psychologist, in 1977 and published in *Psychological Review*,[8] it's lauded as the premier theoretical model for sustainable behavior change.

"Planning creates familiarity, predictability and control," sport psychologist Jim Taylor told me. "All are essential for self-confidence." And self-confidence is critical to sticking with a fitness regimen.

Self-efficacy dictates you find a gym you like—one that's convenient and has a crowd and staff you mesh with. You buy some decent gym clothes you feel good in and hire a qualified trainer to show you the ropes. You feel more confident as you learn and progress at the skill of lifting heavy things and putting them back down. As a result, you're far more likely to stick with it.

Or perhaps you don't go the gym route at all. Through research, experimentation and learning, you figure out something else that tickles your fitness fancy, such as swimming laps, or mall walking, or mountain biking, or whatever. Self-efficacy is about building confidence instead of being a spaz, because confident people have more fun, which intertwines nicely with . . .

Operant Conditioning / Stimulus-response

If you ever took an introductory psychology course, you learned about the work of B.F. Skinner. He's the guy who determined that there are four types of responses that can follow a behavior (the "stimulus"); the response will affect the likelihood of the behavior occurring again in the future. Those four responses are positive and negative reinforcement, and positive and negative punishment. For our purposes, let's focus on positive reinforcement, as it's the most relevant to fitness.

Positive reinforcement is a pretty basic concept: if you do something and it makes you feel good, you'll do it again.[9] This is why weight loss is such a terrible motivator from a positive reinforcement perspective: the response comes a *long time* after the stimulus. With exercise, there's less wait. You can actually enjoy working out, you can like the social aspect of exercising with friends or family, you can have a sense of accomplishment, or just dig the righteous playlist you put together for your walk.

There is, however, an aspect to operant conditioning to watch out for. It's called "extinction." Sounds bad, and it is. It means that if you don't get your expected reward for a long period of time, the behavior designed to get that reward will stop.[10]

Here's an example of extinction (and my wife knows all about it, so just settle down):

Years ago, two other guys and I took a once-a-week boxing circuit class at our gym. Michelle, who looked like actress Jeri Ryan (she played Borg babe "7 of 9" on *Star Trek: Voyager*), always joined our group to make four. She'd hold the focus pads for us to throw punches at and say, "Come on, give it to me. Harder, *harder!*"

I am not making this up.

Needless to say, we never missed a class. That is, until Jeri, I mean Michelle, stopped showing up. We kept going for a few weeks, hoping she'd be there, but eventually our interest in the class waned and we quit. That's extinction—not getting your expected reward makes you quit. It's why motivation must also be intrinsic. It must come from within.

It is important to note that operant conditioning does not take into account the role of cognition (thinking) in exercise or diet adherence.

Human motivation is more complex than simple stimulus-response.[11] An example of this is people who persist in exercising even though they hate it. Such people are rare, but they do exist.

Planning for the "If-Then" Scenario

Life is going to throw you curve balls; it will seem as if more than your share will be thrown with the aim of derailing your new lifestyle. You must plan how you will improvise, adapt and overcome.

"You need strategies that will allow you to create willpower on the spot," psychology professor Peter Gollwitzer told me. One such strategy is the if-then planning mentioned earlier: *"IF* situation X is encountered, *THEN* I will perform behavior Y."* If-then planning can target a temptation in order to avoid a crisis or spell out how to deal with one.

I have an if-then scenario for running. I always have deadlines looming. There's always more writing to be done. Sometimes it's hard to pull away from my damn computer. I hate my computer. My nickname for it is "you stupid @#^$%%*&@%&%!!!"

But "if" I find myself making those "I have so much work to do" excuses to avoid running, "then" I implement this strategy: *just get dressed*.

I pick out the best running clothes I have, admire their quality for a moment and get my gear on, including those $15 socks that are *only* comfortable for running. I even put on my expensive running shoes.

It takes just minutes of motivation to get suited up. Then I go back to my computer and do more work. It generally doesn't take long before I'm out the door.

If-then planning applies to both exercise and food situations. You can imagine dietary sabotage like doughnuts brought to the office, child-care issues with working out, a friend who bails on driving you to Pilates class, an alarm clock that didn't wake you for your morning run, your favorite elliptical not being available, the indoor cycling class being full, Christmas parties or dinner at an Italian grandmother's house . . .

These are all examples of the "ifs" that life can (and will) throw your way. Your job is to strategize a "then" for each and every one. You'll learn how to handle some of them as you go, and you'll develop new and better coping mechanisms over years of practice. Some examples: "if" the alarm goes off and instead of getting up to work out I swear like a sailor for a moment and go back to sleep, "then" I will do my workout at lunch. Or, "if" there is no child care available, "then" I will incorporate my kids into my workout. Your plan can be something concrete—how to deal with certain "ifs"—or it can be as simple as engaging in positive self-talk to get through the challenge so your response eventually becomes automatic.

Gollwitzer says it's important to mentally link instrumental, goal-directed responses to these situations. In English: keep your eye on that prized body. "The stronger the link, the stronger the effect," he told me.

STAY MOTIVATED

Enough academic psychoanalysis. I think I developed an aneurysm writing all that, so let's dumb things down.

At the most basic cognitive level, there are three different motivating forces for human behavior: fear, duty and passion. Sometimes people progress through these three in stages, but not always. Also, they're not all created equal. Let's start with . . .

Fear

This is the least effective motivator and can only work short term. Think of this: each day you go to the gym, you say to yourself, *I have to keep working out or I'll die.* Don't you think that would get old fast? Cardiac rehab programs (you know—people recovering from a heart attack who may die if they don't change their lifestyle) have low adherence rates for this reason. Still, fear can be useful for getting you started.

"Fear was definitely a motivator to get started because my blood pressure was so high," Jane Schmidt, a 47-year-old in Saskatchewan with two grown children, told me. "My doctor got serious on me, and I decided this was it. It was definitely done in baby steps."

And the benefits can kick in fast. Many people will experience a sense of relief that they're finally doing something about their health; the decision to exercise relieves stress.[12]

Sean Astin was referred to as "fat hobbit"—with additional lisping pluralization by the creature Gollum—in his role as Samwise Gamgee in the *Lord of the Rings* trilogy. But did you know Astin runs marathons? I met him the day before we ran the L.A. Marathon in 2012—his third time—and he told me about his battles with motivation and weight, and having an ebb and flow of running adherence. Sometimes he needs to hit a bit of a bottom and have that fear kick him into gear again.

"You're one short run away from feeling like you're moving in the right direction," he told me. "Something about the blood moving makes you feel better." The fear is alleviated because you know you're doing the right thing.

Duty

Duty works well in short and moderate terms. It's your sense of duty that kicks in when you feel you must be healthy in order to be a capable wife/husband/mother/father (or even employee). You realize you can't help or look after people if you're tired, sick or dead, so you pursue fitness to fulfill your duties. Looking at your kids lying asleep in their beds gives you a frequent reminder of these duties, so this motivator works better and longer than fear. In essence, duty can bridge the gap between fear and passion as motivators.

Schmidt's fear transitioned to a duty . . . to herself. "I had always put everyone else first and myself last. It's the mom syndrome. It got to the point where I couldn't sit on the back burner anymore." As it turned out, everyone was supportive of her efforts.

Passion

I've drilled into your head that passion is necessary to succeed. The *Lose It Right* approach is focused on its development. People who are in great shape don't see exercise as a means to an end.

"I went from hating exercise to loving it," Susan Sadler told me. "As a child I had my parents write a letter to my high school to get me out of gym class." If my parents had gone for it, I'd have tried the same thing. "For me, patience was the key. I just took it one day at a time, making small changes that I was able to sustain." Now, Sadler is in the best shape of her life.

And though it's rare, exercise can become such a passion that it leads to significant weight loss all on its own.

"I lost 100 pounds strictly by exercising," Stacy Lynn Carter, a 37-year-old administrative assistant in Halifax, told me. "I ate crap the whole time I was losing weight." Exercising hard up to six days a week dropped the pounds, but Carter admits that then she had to change her diet to keep the weight off.

"Exercise is a passion for me now," she said. "It's hard to hold me down."

You've got to look at this from a "rest of your life" perspective. When you're rushing toward some dropping-weight-for-high-school-beach-reunion-vacation goal, you lose all perspective about enjoying the journey you're about to embark upon. Let's get one thing straight: *it's all about permanent lifestyle change.*

And if you hate it, it won't be permanent.

I will repeat this ad nauseam until it sinks in: you must feel the love. You must take this slowly and steadily and focus on enjoying your new lifestyle, embracing every bit of positive reinforcement you can muster to become a health-conscious workout warrior. Once you achieve this, you'll never want to go back.

Be ambitious. Push your limits slowly, but push them, dammit! See the rest of your life as a series of adventures, a series of quests and physical aspirations. Aspire to live to 100. Aspire to be a fast runner. Aspire to be strong and flexible and agile. Aspire to achieve your genetic potential.

Aspire to be awesome.

8

GET READY: MANAGING TIME, MONEY AND SOCIAL SUPPORT

It takes as much energy to wish as it does to plan.

—ELEANOR ROOSEVELT

It's an axiom in the business world that if you fail to plan, you can plan to fail. Achieving fitness, health and weight loss is no different, which is again why I don't advocate the "just do it" mentality.

"Advance planning is essential to getting in shape," says Jim Taylor. "It creates a mind-set of commitment and it creates the process. Without those, it's not going to happen." Taylor, a San Francisco–based expert in sport psychology who has consulted for elite professional and Olympic athletes, states that most people approach getting in shape without a proper plan, and are hence doomed to fail.

"After six months, half of New Year's resolutions have gone by the wayside," Taylor told me. "And after a year only about 10 percent have stuck with it because there is not a lot of planning behind it."

And according to a 2012 study by researchers at the School of Public Health from the University of Minnesota and published in the *International Journal of Behavioral Nutrition and Physical Activity*, higher use of strategizing for weight control led to better outcomes for improving diet, exercising and losing weight. Those who rarely planned exercise, for example, burned half as many calories per week via physical activity as those who were frequent planners.[1]

So it's time for James to show off his MBA. Here are a few things you need to do to get ready. This isn't the actual exercise and diet plan yet. This is the pre-exercise and diet plan plan. *(Screw you, spell check. I did mean to write plan twice.)* I told you this was more complicated than "eat less, move more."

TIME MANAGEMENT

I've read a lot of fitness surveys, and I can tell you that the number one excuse people give for not exercising is *lack of time*. I'm certain that lack of time has been a boon for the fast and prepared food industries as well. What it means is that people are allowing work to run and ruin their lives.

I'm not going to preach a bunch of time management theories. Several books have been written on this subject; some of them are okay, others not so much. To be honest, I'm dubious about it as a discipline. For me, it's aligned with what I call "self-help bs."

A former employer of mine had a policy that all executives had to take a well-known two-day self-help course on being exceptionally productive through adopting a (lucky) number of mannerisms. I'm being somewhat vague because I'm going to slam the course now. It was the most mindless drivel I'd ever been exposed to. Two days of having common sense you should've learned by age six twisted and paradigmed and proactivated into management mumbo jumbo until my brain turned into protoplasm. Then they try to sell you day planners and software and . . . and just barf. I'm skeptical about whether a time management guru ever helped anyone manage time better. Nevertheless, I didn't want to crap on the entire industry after taking just one course, so I read a couple of the most popular time management books on the market. They confirmed my suspicions that this is common sense overcomplicated so someone can sell a book or a course, along with a bunch of add-ons.

Anyway, I guess I can't just rant about how it's all a bunch of fluff and not give you any advice at all, because that wouldn't be productive, so here is my common sense–based time management advice.

Prioritize

When it comes to time management, nothing is more important than prioritization. Another oft-used axiom in business is that if everything is a priority, nothing is a priority. You must decide that getting in shape is important to you and that you will put it before many other things. It is said that no one lies on their deathbed wishing they'd spent more time at the office. But I think there are plenty of people who lie on that same bed wishing they'd spent more time taking care of themselves, especially since, if they had, they wouldn't be dying right then.

Jenna Lee is a national anchor for the Fox News program *Happening Now*. I spoke to her as things were heating up for the 2012 American presidential election, and even though work was chaotic, this triathlete still found time to exercise.

"I've always found that no matter how crazy the schedule is, exercise has to be a priority for myriad reasons, including the vain ones, but also the health ones," Lee told me. "I never let anything get in the way of exercise."

And it's important to take some "me time" as well.

Jen McKinnon has four children. "After the third kid I didn't bother doing any kind of exercise," she said. "It was too hard. Women have an issue with doing things for ourselves. We feel like we have to martyr ourselves."

By deciding to make holes in her schedule to exercise—taking her "me time"—everything in McKinnon's life changed for the better; it even made her a better mom by making her more energized and less stressed out.

Speaking of which, time management does not just mean making time for exercise. It also applies to making time to eat properly. You have responsibilities in your life, but you have to make the decision that it's okay to put yourself first sometimes. If you don't look after yourself, who will look after your family when you die young? Also, being in great health can make you more productive at everything else you do, including looking after those you love. If you make exercise and healthy eating a high priority, you'll find the time to do it.

One way to find that time is to take it out of TV (or the Internet).

The A.C. Neilsen Co. reports that the average American watches more than four hours of TV a day.[2] According to Statistics Canada, up north we're closer to three hours a day.[3] Either way, THAT IS A MEGA-BUTT-LOAD OF TV!

There's a lot of wiggle room for the average North American to cut into these brain-rot sessions to make time for exercising and preparing healthy meals. Would you really rather keep up with the Kardashians than sweat?

Adapt

Does this even require explanation? This is the "if-then" planning we discussed earlier, because things don't always work out the way you plan, so don't give up on the fundamental goals—just change the plan and try again. Jenna Lee doesn't always get the time she needs for a full workout, so if she has only a short time, she'll crank out a quick 30-minute exercise session and then shower just from the neck down so she doesn't have to redo her hair and makeup.

And my friend Barney Barnowski, a 41-year-old father of two with a demanding job in the technology sector, decided that the only time he was going to find for weightlifting was late at night, so he built a home gym.

"It's more convenient," he told me. "Quite often I will do my workout after the kids are in bed."

Be Efficient

Thirty minutes of going hard with weights is better than an hour of farting around in the gym. Running hard for 30 minutes burns more calories than walking for an hour; it's also better for your heart, lungs and cholesterol. Leaving your front door and running outside takes a lot less time than driving to the gym to run on a treadmill. You get the idea.

Walking and running are two activities that require almost no preparation and can be done anywhere. They are efficient. I have to drive my kids to a one-hour karate class three times a week. Once I actually

nd while you're at it, try to embrace being a "good enough" cook.
on't have to spend hours cooking every day. I'm the cook in our
, and I don't spend that much time at it. There are simple and
y things you can make that everyone will like that don't take a ton
paration time or cost much. Sure, I cook big meals sometimes, but
y doing it when I crank the stereo, crack a beer and have some fun
ping up something healthy and tasty.

It Comes to Exercise, Earlier Is Often Better

later in the day you push your exercise session, the more likely
re to bail out and instead plow butt-first into a Doritos-covered
h.

arbara Brehm is a professor of exercise and sport studies at Smith
ge in Northampton, Massachusetts, and in her 2004 book *Successful*
s Motivation Strategies she outlined how self-control is a limited
rce and that the stress we experience during the day erodes our
ower to exercise. "People who exercise early in the morning have
ighest adherence rates; they have not yet expended time and energy
:oming the barriers that inevitably develop during the day," she
s.[4] I've had a number of email and phone conversations with Barbara.
 cool.

And I can vouch for what she writes. Back in the bad old days when I
n office job and my boss was doing her Donald Trump impression,
 more interested in hitting the liquor store on the way home than
ym.

Chris Shandley is a 43-year-old father of three in Philadelphia, and
 one busy dad. "I just don't have time after work," he told me. "It has
ppen in the morning because there simply is no other time." From
tivational perspective, he likes the fact that he's in the gym almost
:e he's made the decision to be there. "I'm there before I have a
ce not to go. I don't have any excuses."

t may not work with your schedule, and it doesn't mean you're
ned if it doesn't, but this is one powerful adherence tool. Figure out
 works for you, and go with it.

get them there, I've got an hour to kill. Regard
always suited up for a run. As I leave, I see ma
in their cars, reading the newspaper and eating
same types of people who say they have no tim

You don't need a gym, you can go out yo
walk or run on vacation or during business 1
new territory, kill time while the kids are at th
soccer practice. The ways to insert walking an
life are endless. They are the best exercises for 1
that I know.

Running is physically demanding, and beca
back with tremendous results, but this doesn't n
awesome. Walking is the number one form of
More people do it for fitness than anything els
many health benefits. Remember, burning calori
thing in all this. If you like to walk, then walk.

Buy a Slow Cooker (and Some Glass Lock Container

Consider this the "be efficient" section on the eat
slow cooker, I can get a healthy stew, curry or sc
45 minutes flat. I can do the prep the night befo
in the fridge, then plop it in the slow cooker w
controlled and preservative-free dinner is ready
that evening, and there are two or three more ba
feed all four of us—that I can put in Glass Lock a

This is important. Having a few frozen slow-
to prevent eating out. I know the thought proces
out. I don't know what to make tonight. I don't want
don't feel like cooking . . . I have freakin' been there
or the drive-through to the rescue. Well, if you ha
slow cooker in the freezer, it can go straight into
only have to scoop it out onto plates. If you feel a
it on rice. Throw a bowl of grapes on the table a
You go buy one. Buy a big one.

Cathy Beddia did just that. The 39-year-old works at a pharmaceutical company in Montreal; she organized her schedule to make time for exercise. "I picked lunchtime because that was the only time I could do it and stick with it," she told me. She had to talk to her boss about this and get some wiggle room for a longer lunch break, but she found that as long as she put in the required hours, management was cool. And spending her lunch hour working out means she has to bring a lunch instead of eating out. "The exercise definitely reinforces the better eating," she said.

FINANCES

Getting in shape isn't free.

Gym memberships cost. Slow cookers cost. Workout clothing and shoes cost. Personal music players cost. Good personal trainers and registered dietitians cost a lot.

It's all worth it.

I'm not saying you should let your kids starve or send them to raid the lost-and-found bin at school for clothes, but putting some resources into your quest for better health and fitness is one financial investment you won't regret.

Think of it this way: this is your new hobby, and hobbies cost money. This is not some pain-in-the-butt endeavor that's just going to suck dollars out of your wallet; it's something awesome that you like spending money on. Do you play golf? Think about how much that costs.

Compared with golfing, getting in shape should be affordable. Also, if you do eat out or order in a lot, you're probably going to save money on that side of things. As *New York Times* food columnist Mark Bittman pointed out, it's a myth that junk food costs less than real, healthy food.[5] Booze is expensive too. If you cut down on the restaurant eating and give your liver a break, it should even accounts.

Following the advice in this book is more or less certain to help you achieve the following goals:

- Better-looking
- Healthier
- Higher performance
- Improved feelings of wellness and boosted self-esteem

Those things are pretty awesome all on their own. However, recall what I wrote in chapter 3 about how a higher state of wellness can do other things too, like make you more successful in your career. Also think about the sense of accomplishment you'll have. I have reported time and again that getting in shape is not an easy undertaking. By succeeding at this, you'll have a strengthened will to succeed in other areas of life. It is possible that getting in shape will give you the determination to go after and achieve a big promotion, or perhaps launch your own business. You never know, this may end up being the catalyst that makes the rest of your life much more successful.

Shopping! Hooray!

Building self-confidence prior to engaging in a new physical activity helps you persevere.

If you dig up your ratty old sweatpants from high school, put on a paint-splattered T-shirt with a big hole in the armpit, lace up some worn-out tennis shoes and then go for a run, that run is going to suck. But if you go to a running store, get professional help in picking out shoes that are right for your foot shape and your stride and purchase clothing that's comfortable and looks good, you're going to feel a lot better about your first outing. The same is true for any activity, so start planning with care what your chosen activities will be, and get yourself appropriately outfitted. This is money worth spending.

It doesn't have to be a lot of money. If you start with just walking, it can be no money at all. Additionally, you could google "body weight exercise videos" and also spend no money. Beyond that, the only advice I can give is not to financially overcommit to anything. If it requires expensive equipment, try renting first to make sure you like the sport. Try drop-in classes/passes before buying a membership at a club. When it comes to running, start with shoes and socks, and build your wardrobe from there as your passion grows.

When you're starting to form a habit, when you begin to feel the desire to get better and better at something, that's the time when you'll be ready to prioritize more of your paycheck toward it.

Spending Money = Self-efficacy

I've peddled the self-efficacy theory like a Kardashian flogging a fake wedding. Now I want to give you a personal anecdote showing what it means to me.

I'm not just a runner, I'm a Canadian runner. Who hates treadmills. Think on that.

I run outside year-round. I remember running a 10K in hideous below-zero temperatures in an attempt to impress my wife. I ended up finishing in a panic, worried that I'd frostbitten a sensitive part of my male anatomy. That sordid tale was the first fitness article I ever had published, which tells you something about my writing career.

Now I have thermal underpants. They cost $35 a pair.

And a pair of thick running tights that are like pulling on a wetsuit. They do make my butt look good, though. Cost: $95.

My thermal running socks were $16.

On a super-cold day I'll wear a few layers of long-sleeved running shirts. They're all high quality and come in together at around $200.

My gloves have a wind-stopper cover and were $60, but there was a sale and I got them half price.

I have a nice running jacket. I look *good* in it: $100.

I have three different toques depending on temperature, but when it gets Russian-winter-killing-the-invading-army kind of cold, I go for the balaclava. Cost: $22.

The running shoes were $140, and we finish things off with the iPod Shuffle at $50. Grand total of all this gear for one run is $688. Plus tax.

It can be cold enough to have to chisel your dog off a fire hydrant, but to me it's like a challenge issued. Once, on a particularly frigid day, I took all the gear on the above list and laid it on the floor, then took a picture and posted it to Facebook, telling people I was suiting up for a run. There was an equal mix of encouragement and "Are you friggin' nuts?" in the comments. This made for some theory of planned behavior and extrinsic positive reinforcement thrown into the mix for additional motivation.

I've run in extreme cold enough times to learn what clothes I need for what weather conditions. I have a cell phone and emergency Mylar blanket in my pockets, and my wife knows where I'm going and when I'll be back.

Because I have all the gear for cold-weather running, and the experience with using it, I have something else too: confidence.

I know I can handle it, and it's an ego boost. Doing something most other people won't do because it's difficult makes me feel good. The hot shower afterward makes me feel good too.

All it takes is a little cash, wisely invested, to get an all-important confidence boost.

SUPPORT STRUCTURES

There are benefits to going public.

Beyond the managing of time and financial commitment, a lifestyle overhaul requires support. Lots of it. That support can come from a spouse, an encouraging work environment, friends, workout partners, instructors and trainers, even your children.

These people can be a cheering section, or just do things to make your life a little easier, things that allow you the time you need to engage in this transformative process.

Significant Others Are Significant

A significant other can be an important part of your support structure. This is the person you spend most of your leisure time with, after all. If you used to park yourself on the couch every night and watch three hours of reality TV, and are about to give that up for workout sessions and fitness classes, you're affecting his or her life as well. You need to fill that person in on your plan and, if possible, get them onside. Does your partner already exercise? If so, he or she will understand and be encouraging of your efforts. Depending on what they're into, you may even want to exercise with them. Be careful about this, though; what works for them may not work for you. Do your research and don't try to fit into another person's mold.

If they aren't into exercise, your attempt to get more active can be a great motivational tool for both of you to start doing it together. They may not want to start, however, and that's okay. Just don't allow that to derail you in your efforts to get in shape. Instead, be a role model. I was a fitness role model for my wife for 10 years before she caught the bug.

On the healthy eating side, things can also go either way. If you run the show when it comes to meal prep, this makes things easier. Discuss with your partner your desire to begin eating more mindfully, then take the gradual changes outlined in Stage III to make incremental steps toward healthier eating.

But if your significant other is in charge of the groceries and cooking and prefers unhealthy eating (and is not eager to change), you have a problem. This isn't a relationship book and I'm no expert in such counseling, but I can give you some basic advice on this subject:

- Talk to your partner about your need to switch to healthier eating. Make this about you. Don't bring up your spouse's eating habits, weight or health. Chances are they know all about their own bad habits; they don't need you to get all self-righteous on them. Appeal to the fact that they care about you and want you to be happy. Tell them this will make you happy.
- Assure your partner that you don't need to adopt 100 percent healthy eating habits overnight. That can be intimidating for anyone, never mind someone who's less than thrilled at the idea of change. Follow the process of gradual adoption outlined in this book.
- Get involved in the process. Help with grocery shopping, menu planning and cooking whenever possible. If your partner is hesitant about you horning in on their territory, start slow, perhaps

with a night or two a week. Or maybe they'd prefer you to suggest recipes and leave the cooking and prep to them. Whatever works.

The best-case scenario is that your partner may decide to hop on the healthy eating train. If so, this whole thing just got a lot easier. Now you're in this together.

And if children are part of the equation, be sure to check out appendix C for information on making them part of your exercise and healthy eating lifestyle.

Create Positive Peer Pressure

Clara Hughes has won six Olympic medals. I remember hearing her on the radio once talking about how, when she is traveling, she will call friends in various cities in advance to book going for a run with them. She said having that pressure of a friend waiting prompted her to show up.

I interviewed Clara when she was inducted into Canada's Sports Hall of Fame.

"I was very fortunate to be on the receiving end of great extrinsic motivation," Hughes told me. "My coach created an environment where teammates could feed off each other's energy."

I know a lot about this. For years I worked out in a crowded gym surrounded by people I knew and enjoyed being around. I was part of a lunchtime crowd of guys who went to lift weights every workday, and it was awesome. Our raunchy locker-room talk was often the best part.

"Human beings are wired to be in groups," said Bert Carron, a professor of kinesiology focusing on sport psychology at the University of Western Ontario. "Exercising alone doesn't work for the majority of people."

The type of people you exercise with makes a difference. "Birds of a feather like to flock together," Carron told me. "Geriatrics don't want to exercise with a bunch of 20-year-olds, and vice versa. But all of them want to be in a group."

You'll likely want to avoid muscle heads with neck tattoos. Unless that's your thing.

Carron was co-author of a 2006 analysis on the effectiveness of interventions to promote physical activity; it looked at 44 studies, containing 4,578 participants, that lasted anywhere from fewer than three months to more than a year. In the analysis, which was published in the journal *Sport and Exercise Psychology Review*, Carron and colleagues examined the effect on adherence of a variety of exercise scenarios.[6]

Because they were looking at numerous studies pooled together, they measured adherence with something called "effect size," which I had no understanding of, so Carron had to spell out the bottom line in plain English. "Those who exercised alone at home had the lowest adherence rates by far," he told me. "Comparatively, those in the 'collective' group had much higher adherence." When I asked him how *much* higher the adherence rates were for collective groups, he said he measured "a substantial effect. It represents a very large difference."

Carron and I discussed how even if you go to the gym solo to work out, the experience would be akin to being in a group: you're surrounded by fellow exercisers with similar purpose and you see a lot of the same people and even make friends there. So the gym experience would have similar adherence rates to working out in a group. I know the idea of being around like-minded people has pushed me to go to the gym and, once there, stay and get it all done.

Not long ago I made the transition to a home gym, partially for time reasons, but also because I realized the gym I'd spent the past year at was rife with unethical personal training sales practices I could not help noticing (info on how to avoid this is in chapter 10), and witnessing this harshed up my groove. It was a challenging transition, but cranking up the tunes on T-Rex-sized speakers loud enough to make For Sale signs start popping up around my neighborhood made it more appealing. iPods are lame.

I digress. Just know that after 19 years of being a gym-goer, I switched to lifting weights at home alone. Some days, you can hear the Rush from down the street.

For some, exercising at home works. For most, the more Borg-like the "collective," the better.

"It's consistently the same group of people coming to my classes," Chelanne Murphy, who teaches indoor cycling and circuit training classes at World Health Club in Calgary, told me. "Some of the people have been in these classes for 10 years and have developed close friendships as a result."

You will be assimilated. Resistance is futile.

"Never underestimate the power of social support," professor of epidemiology Bill Kohl told me. "It's critical." The more of a situation you can create where people rely on you to be there, or will at least give you some grief if you don't show, the better.

There have been Sunday mornings when I've wakened to a screaming alarm clock with a beer-to-blood ratio that was not conducive to running, and yet knowing my friend Peter would be waiting for me made me drag my butt out of bed, suit up and suck it up. I'd never have heard the end of it otherwise.

The Four-legged Motivational Force

Now don't just go out and buy a dog as if it's a Bowflex. You can't cram the poor thing into the corner and use it as a coat rack. You've got to be a good human. If you are a good human, dogs can be terrific motivators to go outside and get moving.

"The dogs absolutely played an important role in developing my exercise habit," *Dog Whisperer* Cesar Millan told me. "If I sleep in, at 5:15 I start to hear the howling. It's like, 'AARRROOOOHHH! Cesar! It's time to go!'"

Millan says dogs feel as though they're unemployed, and exercise for them is like a job, one that they want to do. "It's a fulfillment and a way of bonding," he said. "A lot of people see dogs just as companionship, but they can also see him as a personal coach and a friend you work out with." (More details on how to exercise with a dog in chapter 11.)

Technical Support

You now know how powerful social support is, but real friends aren't always around to support you. When this happens, the Internet can work well for providing a motivational group hug. Facebook and Twitter are popular, and I've heard of, but not used, a website called Fitocracy.

There are a variety of groups out there that create online social support for exercise adherence, but be warned that such groups are also rife with *terrible* advice about weight loss, diet and exercise. Use them for motivational support, yes, but be cautious about listening to Internet "experts." Bovine droppings abound.

Motivation can be as simple as posting on Facebook about the exercise you've done. My friend Kris, whom you'll read more about in chapter 13, often asks for motivation on Facebook. Encouragement shows up in the comments, and it always gets her moving.

And your fitness friends don't need to be carbon-based. Mobile apps are plentiful for getting you to move (and eat better), though the jury is out about how effective most of them are. Perhaps more motivating are things such as pedometers, heart-rate monitors and GPS devices, all of which allow you to support yourself by keeping track of your performance.

In chapter 7, I spoke of keeping track of *important* numbers, including miles run, lengths swum, weight lifted, etcetera. I also advised paying less attention to numbers on the scale, because it's a damn liar.

The key with record keeping is more about the fact that you keep track rather than what you keep track of. People who keep an exercise log are more likely to succeed long term, regardless of the content of the record keeping.[7]

"I noticed a slow and steady progression in terms of what I was capable of," Susan Sadler told me. "I noticed I was getting stronger, more competent and faster. I've become big on tracking data. I plan every workout. This has been instrumental in terms of my motivation in learning to love exercise," she said. "I fill up notebooks."

Tune Up Your Workout

I know people who are incapable of running without their iPod. I used to be one of them. If the battery was dead, so was my motivation to run.

"These are a class of tools called disassociation," James Annesi, an exercise adherence researcher and director of wellness advancement at YMCA Metro Atlanta, told me. "You're using things like music and television to distance yourself from the discomfort of your workout." What happens with new exercisers, he said, is that they wish to avoid adverse feelings, and something like listening to music can disrupt the negative sensations they feel.

I still listen to music often while running, and blast my stereo while in my home gym. But once I got into training for races, I learned that you need to be in "an associative state" in order to embrace the pain (or something like that). When I'm training hard to make a certain time, I ditch the music because there's no fear of running boredom when you're pushing to the wall.

But the situations in which music hinders performance are rare. It's only for extreme effort that it can get in the way. For the majority of people, music creates a tremendous motivational benefit to their exercise regimens.

Just be careful not to crank it so loud that you go deaf.

A MESSAGE FROM THE DYING

After reading this chapter, you may think this all sounds like a lot of work, and you'd be right. Living a healthier life involves a shifting of priorities, but let me tell why you should absolutely want to make that shift.

Bronnie Ware worked for years as a nurse for the dying. The top two things dying patients said were that they wished they had lived a life truer to themselves (rather than to what others expected), and that they wished they hadn't worked so hard.[8]

George Carlin once said something that covered similar territory: "Life is not measured by the number of breaths we take, but by those moments that take our breath away."

So think about this: You could be breathing in and out working on an expense report, watching TV or doing email. Or you could hike to the top of a hill with someone you love to see what's on the other side, only to have your breath taken away. Such moments can define you.

If you're overworked and it's getting in the way of living a healthy lifestyle, it's time to reinvent yourself. This is your chance to be true to yourself and not regret the way you've lived your life. Start working on a plan to change the way you live, where being healthy is your primary focus.

Make it happen, and that deathbed will be much further away. In Stage III, we're going to provide you with the plan for change. The rest of your awesome new life starts now.

STAGE III:
DO

9

INTRODUCING THE VIRTUOUS CYCLE

*There's a difference between knowing the path
and walking the path.*

—MORPHEUS, *The Matrix*

Suffering is not an effective strategy.

How many people wake up on January 1 with a mouth tasting as if they've been French-kissing a komodo dragon and drag their hungover butt to a place they'd rather not be to do some exercise they'd rather not do because it's time to follow through on that New Year's resolution?

The night before, they had a booze-to-blood ratio that would have tranquilized Charlie Sheen, and now they're going to suffer through something they hate and starve their body with some fad diet because *this year* is the one they finally get in shape.

That's a bad plan. Actually, it's no plan. It's white-knuckle fitness based on the "I must endure this torture" mentality that has a higher failure rate than Midwestern girls heading to Hollywood to become stars.

Disgusting similes and metaphors aside, allow me to congratulate you on making it this far. I realize there's a lot of information to digest, and you've already completed significant work to this point. Way back when, I mentioned that you should ignore Nike's advice and instead "Learn, prepare, *then* do it." Well, you've learned and prepared. Now, you're finally ready to do.

But please bear with me just a little longer while I tell you how the Virtuous Cycle fitness and eating plan works.

THE PLAN

It's time to leave the vicious circle and enter the Virtuous Cycle.

Now you know what junk food does to your brain. Now you know how exercise combats the compulsions this creates and can make you crave healthier food. Now you know how to manage your time and be motivated. Ducks in a row, you can now *Do*.

Doing is a three-level process, though as I mentioned in the introduction, you can hold fast after Level 2. Each level begins with an exercise component to strengthen your ability to deal with food and is followed by a diet component that focuses on incremental improvements. Each level is progressive and more challenging than the last, with exercise and diet continually reinforcing each other—creating a Virtuous Cycle—to keep you motivated and on track.

One thing you should know about the Virtuous Cycle is that we kind of made it up. Don't panic. You can't have gotten this far without realizing that there's a lot of science and expert recommendations packed into this book. I've talked to the experts and researched adoption rates for exercise and altering eating behaviors. And I've collected a boatload of anecdotal evidence provided by real people. All of them (including the hundreds I've talked to over the past two decades who weren't specifically interviewed for the book) say the same thing: weight loss is the result of a steady process toward behavior change in which exercise and eating reinforce each other over time. That, in a nutshell, *is* the Virtuous Cycle.

The model we've designed—and are about to walk you through—involves a *suggested method* for integrating exercise and making changes in your diet. And by "suggested method," I mean what I wrote earlier: we made it up.

News flash: pretty much every diet program out there is something that was just made up. We *don't know* the best way to lose weight, and that's why gimmicks that someone pulled out of their posterior sell so well. Remember the publisher's rejection letter at the beginning of this book? Sensationalism is what sells, but we've rejected that to create a program with the highest possible standards of scientific proof backing it up.

The Virtuous Cycle

E
X
E
R
C
I
S
E

Enhances ability to make wise food choices and makes you crave healthy "fuel."

Increases energy and positive attitudes about being active.

H
E
A
L
T
H
Y

E
A
T
I
N
G

The Virtuous Cycle is based on years of experience, interviews, logic, consultations with numerous clients and gut instinct. But it has not been empirically tested, peer reviewed and published in a reputable journal. Still, you have to admit it sounds like a good idea. So try it, and if it doesn't quite work, modify it. You're a grown-up, and you have the ability to adapt. Everyone is different. Some of you will be great at dietary adherence but hate the exercise component, or vice versa. Some of you may have injuries or illnesses that make intense exercise impossible. The key point is to work your own way through these steps, mixing and matching as needed, and achieve your desired *sustainable* outcome.

So let's break this sucker down.

Steps and Stages 101

I just described how the Virtuous Cycle works, but here are some bullet points to represent the various levels with more clarity.

The exercise levels are
- Level 1A: Making Moves (Easy)
- Level 2A: Fitness Focused (Medium)
- Level 3A: Workout Warrior (Hard)

The eating levels are
- Level 1B: Nutrition Newbie (Easy)
- Level 2B: Gastronomically Good (Medium)
- Level 3B: Eating for Excellence (Hard)

Here it is, laid out in handy chart form:

	Exercise Level	Eating Level	Outcome
Level 1A	Easy	No change	Very low
Level 1B	Still easy	Easy	Low
Level 2A	Moderate	Still easy	Pretty good
Level 2B	Still moderate	Moderate	Good
Level 3A	Hard	Still moderate	Very good
Level 3B	Still hard	Hard	Freakin' amazing

Do you see that last column—outcome? That tells you what you can expect during each level in terms of improvements to health, looks, weight loss, physical performance, mood, stress and other psychological aspects.

And yes, those higher-level outcomes do require a higher level of effort. What's more, you'll be battling the law of diminishing returns, which means that the more impressive the outcome, the more substantial the level of effort required.

And one final note on that front: you want to be careful to stick with the slow and steady pace that we're advocating. There is real danger in trying to do too much too fast. If you overtrain, or are too restrictive with your diet, you can actually start to slide backward on the outcome scale. The graph on the next page shows that the law of diminishing returns starts to kick in around a perceived effort level of 5 out of 10. Beyond 9 out of 10, actual harm can be done.

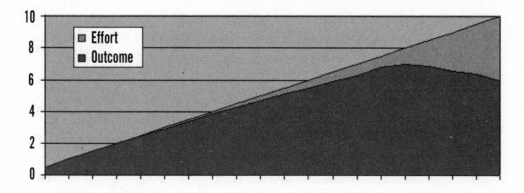

THE THEORY BEHIND THE PLAN

If you're looking at these steps and stages and wondering about our insistence on this slow and steady thing, let me explain again why it's so crucial. Willpower is something that develops slowly. Human beings are creatures of habit, and we can tolerate only small amounts of disruption in our lives without experiencing stress.[1] What's more, psychologists believe willpower is a limited resource. You have a limited amount of energy to spend on self-control. The good news is that willpower is something that can be strengthened with practice.[2]

And practice takes time. Tortoise pacing gives you that time.

Exercise First, Diet Later?

Throughout this book, we've driven home the role of exercise as a powerful tool for dealing with the multiple food temptations of the obesigenic environment. Since we can tolerate only small amounts of disruption, it makes sense to focus on changing just one thing at a time. And Harvard neurologist Dr. Miguel Alonso-Alonso thinks exercise should be first.

"We tend to do exercise and diet at the same time," he told me. "But if we know exercise builds resources to improve diet, why not exercise first to enhance your capacity for eating control and then engage in dietary changes later?"

Why not? We can't think of a good reason why not. In fact, we think it's a brilliant idea.

Why Gradual Exercise Integration Is Recommended

Pain is one big reason why gradual exercise integration makes sense. If you push too hard and too long without giving your body a chance to adapt, you will hate life. No one likes the way it feels to go way beyond her limits, running as if she's being chased by a wolverine coming off a meth bender, lungs rasping like an asthmatic Darth Vader after a dozen bong hits of hydroponic flesh-eating bacteria. Significant results require significant effort, but if you see your dead grandma beckoning you toward the light, you're pushing too hard.

"The biggest mistake people make when starting a fitness program is doing too much and too hard," sport psychologist Jim Taylor told me. "There are few rewards early in an exercise program and many disincentives: a sense of incompetence, negative social comparison, pain, fatigue, sweat . . ."

And if you push too hard, you also may lose *less* weight. This is what a 2012 study out of Denmark found, at least. Using 61 sedentary and overweight men, they compared moderate exercise (burn 300 calories via exercise each day) with high exercise (600 calories per day). And guess what? The "moderate" group lost more weight.[3]

No, I am not gearing up to say "less is more" when it comes to exercise. MORE is more, dammit! However, you need to look at the big picture here. These men were sedentary and overweight. Doing 300 calories' worth of exercise a day did not wipe them out; it energized them. They engaged in additional movement during the day as a result of their moderate exercise regimen, and they also had the brain energy to make wise food choices.

The other group, however, jumped from overweight and sedentary to 600 calories' worth of exercise each day, and this meant they spent a lot of the rest of the day sitting around because they were tired and in pain. What's more, it wiped out the brain energy required to resist eating junk food.

Can you exercise so you're burning 600 calories a day or even more? Hell, yes! But take your time getting there. I go on multi-hour bike rides that burn thousands of calories, but it took me years to develop that kind of endurance. The Danish trial lasted only 13 weeks. Not stopping to carefully analyze the results, as we've done, many in the media (*cough* *New York Times* *cough*) misinterpreted the results as being some kind of metabolic miracle. If the trial organizers had kept the trial going for several months, the higher exercise group would eventually have adapted and most likely become leaner and fitter, but they suffered early on.

Don't make yourself suffer. You'll be less likely to feel the love, and it can hurt your ability to lose weight. You might even injure yourself. Be a tortoise.

Why Gradual Changes to Diet Are Recommended

Back in chapter 1, we recommended Dr. David Kessler's *The End of Overeating* for the way in which it exposes the obesigenic environment. However, we disagree with Kessler's approach to quitting junk food—a total purge of it from your diet, at least until you've gained control over your impulses. "An attempt at moderation won't work," Dr. Kessler says.[4]

We have a problem with that advice.

First off, Kessler quotes only one expert, a professor of psychiatry from the University of Kentucky, who said in regard to eating junk, "It is almost as if there needs to be a total reversal." Beyond that, the majority of Kessler's sources promoting total abstinence studied alcohol and drug addiction, not food.[5]

As we've shown, though it's compelling, food does not meet the criteria to be an addictive substance. Second, you can live without drugs and booze but not food. This obvious fact brings us to *the most important reason why baby steps are key to changing eating behaviors*: it's damn hard, from a practical and time-management perspective, to do an overnight 180-degree turn from a highly processed diet to a healthy one.

Recall that half of American food dollars are spent eating out. *Half!* As we pointed out, a major reason for this is the shift to women working full-time jobs and having far too many time pressures to ensure that every meal has healthy and fresh ingredients purchased from a grocery store and then prepared at home. (Again, we're not blaming women; men did not exactly step up when their significant others took jobs.)

Taking something from box to nuker, hitting the drive-through or order-ing pizza is *so much easier* than actual cooking, and reorganizing and reprioritizing your schedule to accommodate healthier eating will be a lengthy process. From a practical standpoint alone, baby steps trump all or none.

"In my experience a slow and steady approach to dietary changes has been the most successful for achieving sustainable weight loss," obe-sity expert Dr. Yoni Freedhoff told me. Freedhoff also did a thorough review of Dr. Kessler's book for his Weighty Matters blog. His thoughts: "My belief is that the type of blind restriction that Kessler is suggest-ing will ultimately and eventually do exactly what he predicts—magnify conditioned hypereating. Zero tolerance as a dieting strategy has been around forever. If it worked, the world would already be skinny."[6]

"I suggest weaning yourself off junk food," Professor Nicole Avena told me. "I don't think cold turkey is the way to go. Small changes are easier to maintain."

And in regard to the dietary baby steps concept—removing certain bad foods a bit at a time and replacing them with good ones—eating behavior expert Eric Stice said, "This is precisely what we do in our most effective obesity prevention programs . . . I do think this is a better way to get people used to eating healthy foods with few unhealthy foods."

That all being written, if both your schedule and your psyche can handle the complete purging of all junk food without leading to a relapse and/or yoyo dieting, then you go. There won't be (physical) pain or injury, unlike when you go from couch potato to workout warrior overnight. You may find you start losing weight fast, which people *do* like, and you'll start feeling better sooner and be better fueled for exercise.

Again, though, we think the abrupt 180-degree shift is too difficult for the majority of people, so we're sticking to our baby steps recommenda-tion, but it's a *recommendation*, not a law like gravity or thermodynamics.

When it comes to the pace of adoption for dietary change, do what you discover is best for you.

Follow, Bend or Break?

The real reason we're providing these six concrete steps at all is that some people like direct guidance. Whether you stick to the list rigidly or use it just as a general guideline will depend on your personality and your current life situation. So follow these steps, or bend them, or break them if you must. Just follow the basic advice of gradual improvement in both increasing your physical activity levels and eating a healthier diet. You'll reap benefits.

GETTING STARTED

Coming up next is a key piece of the puzzle: a self-assessment to determine how fast you can go through this process, and where you should start. Remember, everyone is different. If you're already active and your diet isn't terrible, you may be able to skip Level 1 and go straight to Level 2. That's up to you. I'm going to be honest with you, though: running the numbers on North American society, it's fair to say about 80 percent of you are sedentary and have lousy diets, so you'll probably be starting off at the beginning. And there is no shame in starting there. Most of the population is in the same boat.

Measuring Your Baseline

How do you know where you're going if you don't know where you start? I know I said I wasn't a fan of the scale, but even if you decide to bury it under a pile of tax returns, it could be good to know where you are right now. Take an assessment of what's important to you, be it weight, waist measurement, endurance, cholesterol or even a "before" picture to go with the "after" you're going to take down the road. One day in the future you'll be pleased with how you compare.

Figuring Out Your Pace

The self-assessment quiz you're about to take looks at your resistance to and ability to change. How you answer the various questions (honesty is key) will help you determine if you should progress through each step at a one-, two- or three-month interval. If you're quick, it will take about six months to become a "Workout Warrior" who is "Eating for Excellence." If you're taking the slow road (again, no shame), it takes 18 months to get all the way through the end of Level 3.

And, yeah, we kind of guessed on this too. There is no hard data on how fast or slowly one should progress through a program like this, but these time periods seem reasonable based on background scientific investigations, our experience and numerous interviews with regular people who changed successfully.

The reason we're being so open about the guesswork is that we're not alone on this front; NO ONE knows with certainty the right way to do this. Beyond the fact that there are no studies showing the perfect way to integrate exercise and change eating behavior, I'll reinforce the fact that everyone is an individual and needs to do some muddling through and finding his or her own way. It's *your* brain getting retrained here.

Look at the bright side: at least we didn't sling a bunch of poop at you—like saying your blood type determines what you should eat—or name the diet after a place where rich people live to make it seem legitimate.

Anyway, when it comes to pace, if you feel that you can *reasonably* go faster, then do. If three months per step is too fast, slow down. If you make it to Level 2 and want to hold fast for a decade before going to the next level, you can do that too. That's what I did. I achieved Level 2 and lost 30 pounds in the process and held firm for more than 10 years; then I upped my game to Level 3 and lost another 20 and have been there another decade.

As I mentioned in the introduction, we're not cracking whips. There is merit in setting goals that are time based, as this boosts adherence to achieving your desired outcome, but this needs to be tempered against the goal of long-term sustainability. Sure, you can kill yourself and get an awesome outcome, but how long can you hang on to that if you hate the journey?

Go at a pace you can tolerate, be at peace, have fun, feel that you're making progress, get all Zen . . . That's a good pace. Sure, do the self-assessment, but do the Zen thing too.

The Self-assessment: How Fast Can You Go?

This self-assessment contains 10 questions. Give yourself 1 point for each "Disagree" that you check. If you "Neither" agree nor disagree, it's 2 points. If you "Agree," it's 3 points.

The lowest score you can get—if you disagree with everything—is 10 points. The highest score, if you agree with everything, is 30.

Get out your pencil and start checking.

Statements	Disagree	Neither	Agree
I have been overweight or obese for many years.			
I work long hours.			
I don't eat many vegetables.			
I spend a lot of time watching TV or on the Internet.			
I am resistant to change. It upsets me.			
My family (spouse and children) is resistant to change.			
My job requires a lot of travel.			
I want to lose more than 60 pounds.			
I eat for emotional reasons (stress/depression/boredom).			
I am responsible for the care of very young children.			
Total number of checks			
Multiply by:	1	2	3
Add these three together for your final score:			

Interpreting Your Score

So what does it all mean? Let me tell you:

- If you score between 10 and 16, proceed through the steps at 1-month intervals.

- If you score between 17 and 23, proceed through the steps at 2-month intervals.
- If you score between 24 and 30, proceed through the steps at 3-month intervals.

It's important to reiterate that *each level contains two steps*. Therefore, the fastest you will progress through a single level is two months, and the slowest is six months. To go through all three levels, following these guidelines, will take between six and 18 months.

If you ended up with a low score, and are looking at proceeding at one-month intervals, it means you're not terribly resistant to change and have the flexibility in your schedule to make it happen. It also means you're likely in a more genetically and psychologically advantageous position to tackle sustainable weight loss.

The folks in the mid range, moving forward at two-month intervals, have a tougher battle to fight, perhaps in terms of genetics, emotional issues, resistance to change or time management. Welcome to the middle of the pack.

For the high-scoring people who are moving at three-month intervals, yours is the hardest battle. You know why. There are cards stacked against you, but do not despair. *When*, not if, you are successful at this life-changing endeavor, you will have developed a set of skills that can be applied to the rest of your life in myriad positive ways. Often it is those who face down the toughest trials who end up achieving the most.

Okay, I have no references to back up that last sentence, but you've got to admit it sounds good.

Enough math; it is time to get your butt in gear.

10

THE VIRTUOUS CYCLE, LEVEL 1

Whenever a thing is done for the first time,
it releases a little demon.

—EMILY DICKINSON

Holy crap, here we go.

I mean, HELL, YEAH! Here we go!

This isn't going to suck as much as you think. Did you see the movie *Castaway*, with Tom Hanks? Remember the scene where he struggled to create a fire from the smallest of embers? Like Tom, you need an ember. You need a small spark of something that you can build on. A good place to start your search, for Level 1, is to experiment and discover an exercise that doesn't suck.

Then you can take that infinitesimal spark of "doesn't suck" and, with time and effort, nurture it into a small flame. With added learning and practice, the flame will become a raging bonfire of exercise awesomeness.

Exercise is cool that way. You can evolve from not hating it, to liking it, to full-blown *Bridges of Madison County* loving it. (My mom made me watch that movie with her. Anything she says about me crying is a lie.)

Enough movie analogies. Let's do this.

LEVEL 1, EXERCISE: MAKING MOVES

This may not be you.

As I mention in chapter 9, you may be at a more advanced stage than this in exercise capabilities (and you may be more advanced on diet as well; one step at a time). However, if you're like most North Americans, easy exercise is the place to start.

Everything you've read here has brought you to this point. We've doomed and gloomed the hell out of you—showing you just how much the deck is stacked against you in the current food environment—in order to convince you that some basic exercise is a critical first step in order to control your desire for salty-fatty-sugary taste sensations.

But now I'm going to tell you that it's okay to decide to make small dietary changes first, and leave beginner exercise for after. We're suggesting exercise first because there is a lot of scientific evidence to support the hypothesis. You know, the stuff we buried you with in chapter 4. However, people are different. If you feel you want to try dietary changes first, go do that. We do, however, encourage you to change only one thing at a time—meaning, alter your diet OR integrate exercise. Both are challenging, and as we've established, humans have limited motivational resources.

Feeling nervous? One day you'll get to look back at what an uncoordinated exercise newb you once were and compare that with how awesome you've become. Keep that in mind. It's a good motivator.

Step 1: Find Your Passion

If you're not active, it's likely because you haven't found your passion yet. Often this discovery happens by accident. As I mention in chapter 4, your exercise soul mate doesn't have to be the best muscle builder or calorie burner. It has to make you happy eventually (don't expect to love a specific exercise right away; many don't). It has to make you want to do it again and again. Finding this soul mate may require playing the field, so to speak. And when it comes to that, Google is your friend. Your real friends are also your friends. Also, don't feel the need to be faithful to any one exercise. In the fitness context, polyamory = cross-training.

Spend some quality computer time researching prospective activities, but don't be afraid to ask friends and family what they like to do. To start things off, here are a few activities I think are suitable for rookie exercisers.

Walking

I am a big, big fan of walking. It's by far the most popular form of exercise on the planet. More people stay healthy via walking than anything else. It's meditative, can be social, is practical and has minimal cost. Plus, you can do it anywhere. Remember chapter 8's discussion of time management? Walking is excellent because it's a great way to kill time if you just dropped the kids off at the mall or some other event, and it's easy to do on a lunch break as well. And you don't need a shower after. All this *and* it gets good results.

Notice I said "good" results. Not great. It takes a lot of walking to burn a lot of calories; the overall metabolic increase isn't that high. As you saw from the chart in chapter 5, running a mile burns significantly more calories than walking it does. What's more, higher intensity exercise does a better job of making the brain changes that lead to improved eating habits. Walking, therefore, is only moderate in its ability to make you a better eater.

That said, if you are sedentary and the only exercise this book gets you to do is regular walking, that's a victory. The health benefits are still significant, so don't discount it.

If you want, it's not a bad idea to get appropriate walking footwear and some good clothes. Take a friend. Walk briskly. Try to get faster. Join a walking clinic. Go farther. Go even faster.

And one day, if you feel you're ready, run.

Weightlifting

I'll give a plug for weightlifting right off the bat. This may seem like an odd activity to recommend for a rookie, but it's a good starter exercise for a number of reasons.

- It is proven to strengthen connective tissues and thereby improve performance and reduce risk of injuries in other activities.
- It can be integrated slowly and steadily.
- It allows you to take breaks, which is a big plus if you're overweight and in poor cardiovascular shape. You lift and you rest. Then you lift and you rest. Over time, you lift harder and shorten those rest periods, but you can start off at a pace you can handle.
- When the fat does come off, you've created an awesomely sculpted body to show off.

What about women and weights?

"One of the main reasons to lift weights is that it's a great way for women to increase self-confidence," Nia Shanks told me. "It's not a perk that comes to mind when they first start strength training, but it absolutely spills over into the rest of their lives." Nia is a strength and conditioning coach in Kentucky, and cofounder of the popular Facebook group Girls Gone Strong.

"I encourage them to use a challenging load of weight," she said. "None of this soup-can-for-500-reps crap. Women greatly underestimate their strength capabilities."

"It ends up changing everything," Jen Sinkler, who until recently was editorial director of fitness content for *Experience Life* magazine, told me. "You might start to get a rounder ass or be able to pick up groceries, but you stick with it because you realize the potential of you. Your emotional and mental strength increase in tandem with your physical strength."

But what about getting too bulky?

"Muscle bulk is dependent largely on testosterone production," Dr. Sue Pedersen, an endocrinologist, told me. "But no woman makes nearly as much testosterone as a man. It really is a hormonal issue. Men have an average of 15 to 20 times more testosterone than women do."

Even if they adopt a hard-core weightlifting regimen, women gain muscle at a comparative snail's pace. For postmenopausal women, whose testosterone levels are even lower, it's even harder to develop muscular size, Dr. Pedersen explained.

"And if you do gain some bulk, it means you're doing good things for your health," she said. Having extra muscle mass helps in injury prevention because the added strength reduces your risk of accidents or falls. "There are metabolic benefits as well. Heavier weightlifting improves insulin sensitivity, so you're less likely to get type 2 diabetes." It's also good for blood pressure control, Pedersen said.

What's more, "loss of femininity is a horrible myth that scares women away from lifting weights," Shanks said. "It's not going to happen. When clients tell me what they want to look like, the images they point to are women who achieved it with a challenging lifting routine."

Sinkler gets the bulking-up question all the time as well. "No one ever became a bodybuilder by accident," she told me.

The Gym Route

As you learned in chapter 8, the social aspect of exercise can be a powerful motivator, so getting out of the house and around other people can help. Even so, not everyone likes the idea. In 2004, the American Council on Exercise surveyed 1,500 people on why they don't go to a gym. The results:

- 46 percent say it's too crowded
- 21 percent say they don't know what they're doing
- 19 percent feel they'll be the only one who isn't "buff or already in good shape"[1]

What are we really dealing with here? When it comes to crowding, I think most of these people are fibbing. In reality, it's an excuse for being intimidated (which is really what the second and third bullet points are all about). Yes, there are times when crowding can be a pain, but this should not get in the way of a dedicated exerciser. I've trained in some of the busiest gyms imaginable, and if you have the right attitude it can feed your energy levels. Empty gyms are boring.

Let's talk about that third bullet point.

There is a chance this is an issue for you. Maybe you're thinking that you don't want to go into a gym full of fit people because you aren't fit.

Some people think they should get in respectable shape *before* they start at a gym so they can fit in better. If you're a big person, maybe you fear others will look down on you.

I don't know how overweight you may be, but I've got something important to tell you about the gym: no one cares.

Seriously, I've worked out in several dozen gyms across five countries and two cruise ships over the past two decades, and I can't think of one single time when I got the impression that an overweight person was looked down on for being there. It never happened to me when I was overweight and first starting. Gyms are accepting environments. If anything, people may see you working hard and think, *Good for him. I hope he succeeds.*

Everyone who works out at a gym knows what it's for. Many there used to be overweight as well. With two-thirds of North Americans being overweight, there's a good chance that a lot of big people are already there (just don't pick one of those bodybuilding gyms where steroid users hang out).

Trust me. Pick the right place and you'll do fine. How do you pick the right place? I'm glad you asked.

The most important things to consider when choosing a gym are location and fit. By fit I mean a place where you feel comfortable; you fit in.

If there's a gym in or near your office building, that's awesome. Community centers are good choices too, and higher education institutions often have gyms that are open to the public.

When you're trying to decide if a gym is right for you, consider things such as who the clientele are (do you mesh with them, or do they make you feel uncomfortable?), hours of operation, change-room and shower facilities, and classes available (more on that below). Take a tour. Ignore most of what the tour guide wants to sell you (especially the personal training—more on that below too) and just look around. If an opportunity presents itself, speak to a person or two taking a break between reps or just finishing on the treadmill. Are they happy? What do they like or dislike about the facility? Don't be afraid to be picky when it comes to this decision, and know you can take time to think on it. In order to make your gym membership worthwhile, this has to be a place you want to come to several times a week. If it's not, you're throwing money away.

Group fitness classes

If you're seriously considering a gym membership, this feature can be an added bonus. Some gyms have great classes, taught by qualified instructors, that they offer at no cost.

If you belong to a decent-sized gym, your menu of choices is likely to include everything from yoga and Pilates to step aerobics, cardio boot camps and Spinning (indoor cycling). Experiment and see what you like. All are great for fitness, burning calories and, most important, for motivation.

These classes create a collective group and can be a place to make friends—friends who expect you to show up again and again and will ask you where you were if you skip. This is positive peer pressure; try to create it.

You can start with beginner classes and up the intensity over time. Spinning classes are a particularly good choice because no one will know if you go easy on the bike tension. As you get more fit over time, you can crank the tension higher and work harder.

Gym-goer Beware
Never let a gym deduct from your bank account. Never give them any banking information at all—not a blank check, not an account number, not even the name of your bank. And be reluctant about recurring credit card payments, as these can be difficult to stop. A better route is to negotiate the best contract terms you can for one year (which many gyms are going to want to lock you into as a minimum time period; you'll pay a premium for going month to month) and then pay the whole year up front, *in cash*. At the end of that year you can walk away if you've moved on to another activity (or to another gym) with no fear of ongoing payments.

Home gyms

I'm about to gently discourage you from going the "home gym" route, for the following reasons:

- There are many distractions at home (partners, kids, television, laundry, telephone, errands, etcetera). And you can consider time away from home at the gym as your "me time."

- As I pointed out in chapter 8, exercise adherence rates are at their lowest for people who work out at home, alone.
- Home gyms take up a lot of space, and they can't rival the equipment in a good gym.

That being said, some of us have brains that are just wired differently. Your life circumstances (babies at home, for example) may make it difficult to leave the house. Or you may live in the middle of nowhere (i.e., a place that doesn't have a decent gym within driving distance).

If you really think that a home gym is the best way for you to go, it's possible to make a small investment in some basic equipment, integrate bodyweight exercises (TRX—google it), get a Swiss ball, dumbbells and some exercise bands and make significant progress. What's more, if you have someone at home to act as a workout partner, it's possible to make the experience even more motivating through a team approach.

A word or three about trainers

I urge AGAINST using any trainer at a franchise gym. I have investigated the personal training industry in depth and learned that these gyms value their trainers' *sales skill* over their abilities as trainers. They have quotas to meet and use high-pressure sales tactics to get you to buy far more training than you need. Two people I interviewed stated that the gyms they worked for focused on pitching an entire year's training— worth around $10,000—to every prospective client regardless of goals and needs. You can use a franchise gym as a place to work out, but I repeat, do NOT use their trainers. You are viewed by management as a cash machine, and once they get their personal training hooks into you, they are loath to let you go.

Motivated yet?

Hey, it's not as bad as it sounds. Just find a good trainer elsewhere (and if you want to work out at a popular gym and need training, you'll have to find it elsewhere; a franchise will not permit outside trainers). There are many trainers who have their own studios, and there are other "mobile" trainers who will come to your house. Whatever route you choose, I recommend that you pick someone with a degree in kinesiology or at least a two-year personal training diploma from a community college. In addition, they should have a quality personal training certification. In the United States, NSCA and ACSM are the best certifying bodies, whereas in Canada it's CSEP.

Also, find someone you like. There should be a good personality fit. Some of us like to be yelled at until we beg for mercy, others not so much. Choose accordingly.

Whether you opt for the home or the traditional gym route, if you have no or little experience, I highly recommend that you consult a trainer. For how long is up to you. Personally, I'd suggest minimizing the total number of sessions for two reasons:

1. You spend less money, and I'm cheap.
2. You develop greater confidence when you learn to go it alone.

That second point is an example of self-efficacy. If you always have a trainer holding your hand, your ability to develop intrinsic motivation to go it alone suffers. A good trainer will help you develop this kind of motivation, but you have to make it clear that this is what you want to do. You have to tell them you want to "graduate" from needing them after about six or 12 sessions (or however many you are comfortable with), so can they please teach you to be independent?

Of course, if your boat is worth more than my house and you can afford some sexy person to motivate you for every single training session from now until doomsday, and if this makes you happy, then go big, but know that a program does not need to be complex to be effective.

"Consistent practice combined with good nutrition and practicing good form and working to fatigue—no matter what the [amount of weight]—is what makes up the majority of results," says Stuart Phillips, a professor of kinesiology at McMaster University in Hamilton, Ontario. "I think a lot of the variables in a resistance training program—rest, sets, loads and other variables—are largely redundant in their capacity to bring about strength and [bigger muscles]." More important to

Phillips is that you "get to the weight room, consistently practice, work to fatigue—this is 80 percent of the job."

Cycling

Zero impact, good calorie burner and lots of fun. It's great to do with the family too. Go for it.

And don't be ashamed to buy a power-assisted bike for the hills. These are becoming more popular all the time and making cycling for fitness more inclusive of people who don't yet have the stamina to handle tough hills. You still get a good, fun workout, but when facing a steep incline you can let the electric motor help you out or even do all the work.

There's a guy in my city in his 80s. He has emphysema from years of smoking, and he can barely walk. But he rides his power-assisted bike all the time. I've seen him out on the paths. He quit smoking 20 years ago and took up cycling, and the motor helps him keep active by doing the parts he's no longer capable of.

If that's not enough of a motivator for you, consider that cycling is also an excellent source of transportation.

"I've always loved cycling," said Eric Goebelbecker, a 48-year-old dog trainer and computer programmer. "New York is one of the most bike-friendly cities in the US. It was a way to make me get 45 minutes of exercise each way. I have a road bike for the nicer eight months of the year and a crappier one with more appropriate tires for the other four months."

Eric had knee surgery a few years ago, and his desire to lose weight was partially motivated by knee issues. Cycling became an obvious choice because running was painful. Now he saves on parking, tolls, the bus and subways, gas, insurance and car maintenance. Also, "driving in traffic sucks," Eric said. Now he avoids that.

Hiking

This is another great activity that has a lot of possibilities for beginners. It can be done with the family in a local area, or you can google your local outdoor pursuits organization and go on a group hike.

And it doesn't have to be just a fair-weather activity. A trip to a mountaineering store can get you outfitted for any and all conditions, even deep snow if you rent a pair of snowshoes.

Swimming

Yet another activity that's good for beginners. A lot of people love this sport, so consider giving it a try.

"Every swimmer I know who has made it big is extremely passionate about the sport," said Matt Grevers, an Olympic champion who attained gold for Team USA in London 2012. "It's not just competitiveness but about loving the sport. It's not about beating someone else but about being the best you can be. Swimming has defined me as a person; I feel like I'm a better person all around because of it."

Matt Grevers really loves to swim. Maybe you will too.

To prepare, all you need is a suit, goggles, maybe a bathing cap, and a pool with lap swim hours that meet your schedule. With the availability of indoor pools, bad weather is no excuse not to go. Check your local recreation center, college or university for a place to get wet.

As you can see, there's no shortage of activities suitable for a person new to exercise. And I'm barely scratching the surface here. You never know what's going to grab your attention and make you want to get up and go. And keep track in this experimentation stage of what works for you and what doesn't. If something isn't working, make the necessary changes. You can adapt.

Step 2: Implementation

Once you've zeroed in on some exercises you want to try, you need to take the final steps toward getting active. This is more self-efficacy stuff: building up your situation-specific self-confidence in advance of the activity. These are things such as more research into your chosen activity, arranging for lessons, checking walking and cycling routes, talking to people who engage in these sports and buying the appropriate gear and clothing.

You also *must* consider the time and scheduling factor. Remember that morning exercisers have the highest adherence rates for regular fitness regimens, so try that. Also recall that the later in the day you push it, the more likely you are to bail and hit the couch (or drive-through) instead of the gym, bike path or pool.

You need to take a close look at how to make adherence happen. Things such as time of day, location, finances, child care, spousal support, gear and more all need to be figured out to reduce stress and boost confidence. Writing things down helps.

So prep first, sweat later.

There's an additional bonus to thorough preparation, and that's the building of excitement. If you're a rookie, consider this: I've just told you *not* to exercise for the next week or so but instead to get ready to exercise. By the time you start, you could be feeling revved up and totally gung ho. Anticipation is a wonderful thing.

Step 3: Form a Habit

You're ready, you're set, now GO . . . form a habit. THIS is the *number one goal* of the "easy exercise" level. The calorie burning isn't that high. The effect on your muscles and health is moderate. The physiological and psychological changes as they apply to eating behavior are also moderate. BUT! You get into a routine. You take those important first steps toward exercise becoming a habit. Even if you never feel the love, exercise can become habit forming. It can become something that you just do, period.

Do you recall, back in chapter 7, our discussion about "if-then" planning? A large part of getting over your unwillingness to exercise (if, indeed, you are unwilling) is about habit formation. Yes, feeling the love for exercise is important, but don't disregard the power of just doing it because it's what you've programmed yourself to do. You may see getting up early to run most mornings with a big smile and saying "I love running!" as an unattainable goal—or masochistic. But it's easier to imagine it becoming something you get up and do when the alarm goes off because you've strategized it into your life as a regular routine and have *just become used to it.*

"The first few months it was a grind, but I had a couple of revelations," Darlene Bordin, a 42-year-old mother of two in British Columbia, told me. "There were times my alarm went off and I decided not to go, and I lay there in bed for an hour. I decided I wasn't going to do that again. The easy part is setting the alarm, and I have never regretted getting up and going for a run, but I always regret not having gone. It's routine now. You just do it. It's like brushing your teeth and taking a shower."

So stick with it. Get used to it. Get a little better at it. Before long it simply becomes a habit.

Step 4: Take Measure

Ever heard the expression "what gets measured gets done"? This is an MBA-ism and I can attest to its veracity.

In previous chapters we learned about research that shows how tracking progress is a proven motivational tool, and we discussed process versus outcome goals. I remind you here to write out your process goals and stick them on the fridge. Seeing them every day, and seeing the progress you're making in achieving them, is powerful.

Many are fans of writing down your outcome goals as well, but I don't see this as necessary. Some will quote the "Yale Study of Goals" to bolster the claim, asserting that in 1953 a Yale graduating class was asked if they had specific, written goals for the future. The 3 percent who did had accumulated more wealth than the 97 percent who did not.

Cute story. And a myth.

The study never took place. It might make a difference to write down your long-term/outcome goals, or it might not. At the very least, get a solid idea of them in your head. That should suffice.

Step 5: Be Ready for the Epiphany

Shinedown singer Brent Smith was on his way down. It was two years after the Kathie Lee Gifford *Today Show* debacle mentioned in chapter 3, and he was in bad health: overweight, eating junk and drinking far too much.

"I'll never forget the day my girlfriend, Teresa, sat me down—it was the first of November—and said, 'Listen to me, I love you and I'm not going anywhere, but this lifestyle that you're leading is not going to work,'" Brent told me. Five days later he was meeting with his trainer for the first time. And he was hungover.

"I was in really bad shape," he said. "I'm five foot eight and weighed 222. Teresa had told me it was time to get my life back. I felt like I'd been in a death spiral, and I realized I needed to be healthy and strong for my family. I have a four-year-old boy and he was a huge motivation, and so were the fans. I had an epiphany working out with my trainer that day, and I haven't had a drink since."

That epiphany led to 70 pounds of weight loss in a year. Walking into that gym, seeing all those healthy people working out, made Brent realize he wanted to be one too.

I've had my own series of epiphanies. The first came when I saw a photo of myself taken during summer vacation. I was fat. It didn't look like the me I was familiar with. I have obesity in my genes and I didn't want to go any further in that direction.

Learning to get good at weightlifting was another, and the first step in becoming fit. Once weightlifting became ingrained into my lifestyle, I began tasting the fruit and vegetable rainbow instead of the Skittles one. I even attempted running. And I hated it, and I quit.

Then I tried running again, and I hated it, and I quit.

Then I tried again, and I hated it, and I did not quit. And one day I was running through horrific weather conditions with sideways precipitation while U2 was blaring on my iPod telling me it's a beautiful day, and I thought, *It sure is.*

Exercise is locked in your genes. We're programmed for it. You've likely buried the impulse deep, but it's still there, lying dormant, waiting to come to the surface.

It doesn't always happen on day one, or even on day 100. But if you're paying attention, if you seek it out, the epiphany that physical activity is something you're born to do will speak to you.

Make sure you're listening.

LEVEL 1, EATING: NUTRITION NEWBIE

There's merit in keeping things short and simple: simple is easier to follow. So I'm going to keep this part as basic as possible while still being informative. You may remember from chapter 9 that the Virtuous Cycle eating plan is built around the concept of replacement. We remove one thing and replace it with another. These replacements are healthier and lower in calories, fuel exercise performance better and are more satiating. And yes, they *do* lead to weight loss. Simple, right?

Unlike the exercise section, this one has no particular order to the advice *within* each diet level. We provide a list of recommendations that may or may not apply to you. Your goal is to tackle as many as you can without getting too uncomfortable. It should be a bit uncomfortable, though.

As you proceed to Level 2 and Level 3, however, the dietary changes will be more challenging. Level 1 features dietary changes that are the easiest to accomplish—not just from a "resisting junk food" perspective, but also from a time management (taking time to cook) perspective. The next levels may be more challenging as the reward value of food declines, as well as in the work required to replace those ultra-delicious "foods" with healthier choices.

Here we go.

CUT Sugared Soda and REPLACE with Diet Soda

I can hear the sharp report of hippie brain aneurysms from here. *Grab your torches and pitchforks!*

Do I think diet soda is good for you? No, I don't.

Do I think sugared soda, sports drinks and energy drinks are light-years worse? Yes, I do. Diet soda is a far lesser evil than any of these. It's like methadone for weaning you off the sugared stuff. If you want to go to club soda or water instead, great. You go. But if you need something sweet-tasting as a replacement to get you off sugared soda, the diet varieties are the way to go. They make kinds now that don't taste like an ashtray.

Now that that's out of the way, let's tackle a few diet soda myths. First, the satiety issue. Some claim diet soda doesn't help with reducing caloric intake because there is a compensatory effect, but Purdue University professor of nutrition Richard Mattes explained that it's all about how you use the drink. "It's not a product of the artificial sweetener, it's more of a cognitive effect. If you think that you've earned more food by drinking diet soda, it's not going to work. You have to make a conscious effort to not go hog wild later on."

Swapping sugared soda for diet is about cutting calories. If you drink two Cokes a day and switch to diet, that's 300 fewer calories you're drinking each day. Don't screw it up by thinking you've earned a food reward.

Second, let's address safety. Is aspartame good for you? Probably not, but all that sugar in regular soda is bad for a lot of reasons too. Ever hear of type 2 diabetes? Yeah, there's that. It's way worse than any potential problems posed by aspartame, which the alternative medicine crowd have blown way out of proportion.

I find it amazing that people will consume large quantities of unregulated and questionable supplements, yet rag on something that has been extensively tested for safety by multiple regulatory agencies.

The most common artificial sweeteners on the market (aspartame, sucralose) are classified as GRAS—Generally Recognized as Safe. The World Health Organization, the Scientific Committee on Food of the European Commission, the Joint Expert Committee of Food Additions of the United Nations Food and Agricultural Organization, and the United States Food and Drug Administration were all involved in granting this classification. The available data about the use of a substance must be known and widely accepted by qualified experts in order for it to receive the GRAS classification. There must be consensus that the substance is safe under the conditions of its intended use. Over 100 regulatory agencies around the world are cool with this stuff in moderate doses.[2]

I read that aspartame can increase the incidence of bladder cancer in male rats, though. Hmmm . . . scary stuff. Actually, if you look at the data, male rats are highly prone to bladder cancer in the first place—it's almost like if you sneeze on the buggers they get it—and they received 100 times the amount any human would normally ingest.[3]

Don't mainline aspartame. Take it easy. Use it to wean yourself off sugared soda, and then wean yourself off the diet stuff too. Water is always your best choice.

CUT Most Juice and REPLACE with Fruit

Juice packs in more calories, has less fiber and is not satiating. So apples, not apple juice. Oranges, not orange juice. Grapes, not grape juice.

Most of the time.

CUT High-calorie Coffee Drinks and REPLACE with Just Coffee (and Maybe Some Milk)

Gobs of cream, lots of sugar, and the Big-Mac-calorie-rivaling unpronounceable drinks need to go. A little 2 percent or whole milk in your coffee to take the edge off is fine.

CUT Stealth Sugars and REPLACE with Unsweetened Foods

I will remind you to google this: "FDA Nutrition Facts Label Programs and Materials."

You need to learn how to read labels. Many of the foods you buy—pasta sauce, soup, corn chips, granola, etcetera—can be loaded with what David Katz calls "stealth sugars." If you check the labels, you'll find them there under "Total Carbohydrates," labeled as "Sugars." Choose items with the number of grams of sugar lower than the other options.

When you switch to unsweetened varieties of various foods (like pasta sauce), you'll barely notice the difference. An added benefit of this approach, says Katz, is that when you remove these hidden sources of sugar from your diet, your sensitivity to sweetness goes up. Therefore, those other sugary treats you consume start to taste a little too sweet. Cutting back on them at a later date becomes easier.

CUT Chips with a Million Ingredients and REPLACE with Chips with Few Ingredients

This is more advice from David Katz, who has written about certain chips being sprayed with a finishing layer of high-fructose corn syrup to make them more irresistible. That is so not cool.

He favors chips that have three ingredients: whole-grain corn, canola oil and salt.

You'll eat fewer of them, and the switch will cut down on your sugar intake (and start retraining your brain to lower your sweetness threshold. Lowering your sweetness threshold is a good thing).

CUT Two Junk Food Snacks per Week and REPLACE with Apples (or Some Other *Fresh* Fruit)

Pretty straightforward. Track this. Plan for it. Shop for it. Work it into your schedule. Be mindful of food.

Do it.

CUT Alcohol Intake by 25 Percent and REPLACE with Water

No explanation required.

That wasn't so bad, was it? That's it for your first dietary step. If you've read through this and are now sitting there thinking that not many of these apply to you, feel free to jump ahead into Level 2. The goal is to get a bit uncomfortable with these dietary changes and work at them until they become comfortable. Then you'll be ready to get a little uncomfortable again.

Don't beat yourself up when you fail (notice I didn't say "if" here; you will slip up—you're human). Everything is a learning experience, and better eating takes practice. Every failure is an opportunity to learn and do better next time.

11

THE VIRTUOUS CYCLE, LEVEL 2

We are what we repeatedly do. Excellence,
therefore, is not an act but a habit.

—ARISTOTLE

Congratulations on making it this far. Don't stop now! While Level 1 can impart solid health benefits, it's just scratching the surface of awesome. Level 2 is where you can see some significant results. As I mentioned, it's perfectly acceptable to make your way through this level and then hold firm. Level 3 is pretty hard-core, and if it's not for you, that's cool. Let's make it through Level 2 and see how you feel.

LEVEL 2, EXERCISE: FITNESS FOCUSED

Many of you are probably trying to figure out just what "fitness focused" means. To be totally honest, it's hard to say. This isn't, after all, an exact science, and much depends on your starting point. Still, I know people like to have guidelines, so I would say that by the time you have yourself well into this step, you should be hitting about three or four hours of exercise a week at a pretty good intensity.

Does this sound like a lot? For a couch potato, I'll bet it does. But there are 168 hours in a week. Four hours a week of exercise equals 2.4 percent of that. It's not so much. It's what the average American spends watching TV in a single day.

So how do you become fitness focused? I'll tell you.

Step 1: Establishment

Once you've found an exercise that's not so bad, you have to make it part of your routine.

You'll have your ups and downs, for certain, but you need to get to the point where you feel you have this down as part of your regular schedule. This is where printing off that schedule and sticking it to the fridge can help.

For those who decide to work out at lunch, I advise blocking off 11:45 to 1:15 in your electronic calendar so people don't book you in meetings that go until noon but somehow stretch to 12:15 and throw you off, or have you dashing to a one o'clock meeting all sweaty and gross. And try to keep track of when you bail and when you stick it out; this information will come in handy as you work to keep this exercise thing going.

For those tackling a workout early in the morning (good for you!), make sure you have your gear ready to go the night before. As soon as that alarm goes off, know that you've got to motivate yourself for only the 30 seconds it takes to get out of bed and start brushing your teeth. Once those vanity lights hit your eyes, you'll be awake, and you won't have anything better to do with the time, so you might as well work out. As an added motivation, have the coffee timer so your first cup is freshly brewed and waiting.

Most important, know that this stage of the Virtuous Cycle is a fragile time, so *focus!*

This is where you build the foundation for changing everything. When you build a house, you start by digging a hole. Then you build forms and pour cement, and it takes quite a while before things even get back to ground level.

Okay, that analogy doesn't make a lot of sense. What I mean is, don't expect to see a lot of *visible* changes just yet. In this stage, your major accomplishment is sticking to a regimen and garnering health benefits. It's not until you put Level 2's dietary changes into effect that you will begin to see a significant change in the mirror (I know vanity motivates, which is why I'm even bringing this up).

You *will* start feeling better and more energized, however, and that's a big thing; it's something to be proud of. Your exercise doesn't have to be super intense, lengthy or every day. It's just got to be regular and not a lame effort.

Again, don't sweat the fat loss aspect so much yet. You're not ready for sustainable fat loss. The reason for this can be described via the old joke that the easiest way to gain five pounds is to lose 20. In other words, lots of people lose 20 pounds and then gain 25 back. I don't want you to be one of those people.

Screw that stupid scale.

My ultimate goal is to have you "transcend" the scale, to have you get to a point where you just don't give a damn about what it says because everything else in your life has become so awesome. I almost never weigh myself, and the only reason we have a scale in the bathroom is because the kids are growing and like to find out how much they've gained, not lost. If it were up to me, I'd shove it in the storage room so I didn't have to keep stubbing my toe on it. Well, we also need it to weigh luggage to make sure we're not over the airline's stupid weight limit when we fly.

The numbers on the scale really shouldn't matter. Scales lie. You could be retaining water or constipated or maybe you've gained muscle. Consider just hiding the damn thing and digging it out for a look only when you're curious because you feel you've accomplished a lot.

In chapter 7, I suggested that belt notches, how pants feel, and the mirror are more accurate indicators of progress. I may never use a scale, but I use that mirror every time I shave to see what my midsection looks like. It beats what any scale can tell me.

Now let's talk about some numbers that do matter.

Step 2: Frequency, Intensity, Length and Difficulty

Level 2 is all about taking what you did in Level 1 and pushing it harder. We're in Stage III, which is *Do* mode, so when it comes to exercise, do it more often, do it harder and do it longer. You can even pick more challenging things to do.

Here is how it breaks down.

Frequency

The number of times you exercise a week; that's a good number to track.

Were you a total couch potato, and now you exercise twice a week? Awesome.

Go for three.

Then four.

You get the idea. You know how this works now.

Intensity

How heavy are those weights you're lifting? How many sets did you do? How fast did you run? What pace did you swim at? How high is the bike tension in the spin class? Lift heavier weights. Run or swim faster. Push harder in your fitness class. Take your chosen activity and just give it more. Your heart should beat faster and your breathing should be heavier. This is about increasing the level of effort.

All these exercises have intensity numbers (tension, speed, weight) that you want to increase, baby step after baby step, tortoise-ing your way to ultimate victory.

And that ultimate victory can translate into other numbers, such as improved cholesterol and blood pressure, lost inches of fat and gained inches of muscle, even gained number of visible abdominal muscles, if you're superambitious.

Length of Time

Perhaps your average workout time was 20 minutes. Now it's time to go to 30 minutes. Then 40.

Work out longer. Run farther. Swim more lengths. Cycle more miles. Then do more.

Experiment with Higher-difficulty Exercise

Remember when I said that total newbs didn't need to adopt exercise regimens that were great calorie burners or wonderful muscle builders? Well, it's time to start changing that.

It's time to start kicking your own ass, just a little.

It's time to embrace the (little bit of) pain. Start trying out the harder stuff. Not running yet? Perhaps it's time. Stuck on a stationary bike? Go outside on a real one and go faster. Lifting weights with machines? Get some good training on the free weights, and maybe try kettlebells. Still taking the beginner Spinning classes? Try advanced. And maybe give power yoga a shot instead of basic.

Start searching for things that burn more calories, demand more of your body, get better results and make you feel that you *carpe*-ed that *diem* a little more.

Remember, it's not just the direct physiological changes you're questing for by pursuing more intense forms of exercise, it's the psychological boost you get from doing so. When you get good at going hard at physical fitness, you build a skill of mental toughness that makes you more capable when it comes to dealing with food. You get that enhanced "executive function" we talked about in chapter 4, which makes you more capable of sticking to a healthy eating plan.

Don't hurt yourself, but don't hold back either. When you progress and give your body time to adapt, you can accomplish amazing things.

Born to Run?

Did you walk in Level 1? Did you try short bursts of jogs? It's time to give this sport a try. I'm going to push this one again, because it's a great example of how pushing yourself can get amazing results. Plus, it doesn't cost much, is a fantastic and practical time saver, and is addictive.

First, though, let's bust some myths about running.

"There is a clear body of evidence that running does *not* lead to the development of osteoarthritis," says Reed Ferber, an associate professor of biomechanics at the University of Calgary and director of its Running Injury Clinic. "Some of those studies have good evidence that it is actually protective of joints."

"There is really no evidence that running causes joint injuries," echoes Irene Davis, an expert in biomechanics and director of the Spaulding National Running Center at Harvard Medical School.

In fact, Davis told me (with apologies to Bruce Springsteen) that humans were born to run. "I think we evolved to run," she said. "It's in our genes and is the most natural exercise we have. It doesn't make sense that it would wear you out."

And being heavy is not an excuse to sit on the sidelines. A 2003 study in the *Journal of Biomechanics* compared knee loading in 21 obese and 18 lean subjects. When the obese subjects walked at their usual (slower) pace, they experienced less knee loading than the lean subjects. When everyone walked at the same pace, the knee loading was also the same. The authors proposed that obese subjects had an "ability to reorganize neuromuscular function" to protect their knee joints.[1] It's possible this could be true for a cautiously paced running program as well.

"I'm sure some obese people do have knee pain because they don't exercise," Ferber said. "Immobilization has corrosive effects for your cartilage. Moving is what lubricates your joints."

Harish Ganesh, 40, is an entrepreneur and father of two living in Kochi, India. Running is what enabled him to lose over 50 pounds and drop his waist size from 38 inches to 30 inches. "Exercise was anathema for me," Ganesh told me. But then he started walking. "Slowly, I was starting to enjoy my walks." His walks got longer and longer, until he became a runner, which changed everything else. "I understood that exercise was motivating me to eat healthily," he said. "Running for me is a passion now." And that's why he's successful at keeping weight off.

"I tried running but it just hurt too much," Jen McKinnon told me. "So I just kept walking and it just kept getting longer and longer. Then I started running bits and pieces during my walks, and now I've got my first 10K race coming up." And like so many others, McKinnon said, "All this exercise has put me in the right mind-set for dealing with food."

Graham Levy is a 43-year-old electronic technician in Halifax who began running in 2010 because a friend was training for a half marathon. "I thought it would be cool," he told me. He started with walking too. The walking led to 40 pounds of weight loss. "And then I got light enough that I felt ready to start running." He's down a total of 65 pounds, and has run his fourth marathon, with his latest effort being under four hours. Now he's got his eye on qualifying for the Boston Marathon.

Anna Mae Alexander is 29 and lives in Calgary. "Three years ago I couldn't walk," she told me, referring to her polymyalgia rheumatica. "I started controlling it with foods that were less inflammatory, then began walking. I worked my way up to doing the 60K Weekend to End Breast Cancer, then registered for a Learn to Run program. I've done a few 5K races now."

If you try to become a runner and fail, don't give up forever. Third time was the charm for me.

Tune Your Technique

When I decided to start training to qualify for the Boston Marathon, I went to see Cory Fagan, who operates TCR Sport Lab in Calgary, to get some coaching. One of the most important things he did was change my running technique. Try these tips to get faster and avoid injury:

- Stand tall and lead with your chest. Imagine there is a string at the top of your head pulling you skyward. Don't slouch forward when you run.
- Fast hands = fast feet. Keep a small angle at your elbow so your thumbs almost brush

Fun with Fido

If you want a dedicated running partner, there are certain breeds of dog that can go the distance, but there are cautions as well.

"For any breed, you want to start out with an exam to give them a clean bill of health," said Idaho-based Marty Becker, the veterinarian for VetStreet.com and author of more than 20 books on pet ownership, including *Fitness Unleashed*, about working out with your dog.

"Wait until the dog is fully mature until you really start pushing the mileage," said Katrina Mealey, a professor of veterinary medicine at Washington State University. And keep in mind that certain breeds of dog are better adapted to running than others.

"Dogs with pushed-in faces—pugs, Pekingese and Shih Tzu, for example—have a hard time breathing normally," Becker said. "If you take them too far or too fast, they are at risk of dying."

Mealey added that these short-muzzled dogs can't tolerate heat as well either.

Some specific recommendations from Becker and Mealey for dog breeds that *are* good distance runners: border collies, German short-haired pointers, Dalmatians, Labrador and golden retrievers, and standard poodles. Even if you want to run sprint intervals, they can keep up.

And the dog doesn't have to be big. Mealey had a Jack Russell terrier that would keep up to her fast pace for eight miles.

your chest as you run. Don't let your arms hang low, but keep those hands high and pump them in short, rapid movements.

- Try to be quiet. Act as though you are sneaking up on someone so that you land soft rather than slam your feet into the ground.

I'll close this section with a reminder. Fitness Focused is about incremental pushing in four key areas:

1. *Frequency* of exercise: Do it more times during the week.
2. *Intensity* of exercise: Go harder, sweat more, get a higher heart and breathing rate.
3. *Length* of exercise session: Make each session longer.
4. *Difficulty* of exercise type: Pick harder classes, go from elliptical to treadmill, run instead of walk, swim instead of aquacize . . .

You don't have to push all four things at the same time, but do keep them in mind. That list you've put on the fridge? Write this along the top: "Remember to push."

The acronym to keep all of this in your head is FILD, because you will feel as though exercise has "filled" your soul.

Gak! Ack! Blarf! My stomach is heaving right now. I can't believe I wrote that. Next section, please . . .

LEVEL 2, EATING: GASTRONOMICALLY GOOD

If you're reading this, I trust you've adopted the Fitness Focused exercise level. That's good, because it's about to get harder, and you need the brain- and will-strengthening benefits of physical activity to power through.

You know how this works. Here we go.

CUT White Flour and REPLACE with Whole-wheat Flour

We're not asking you to cut fast food yet, so you can still have your god-awful McDonald's/Wendy's/Burger King/Arby's buns. For the stuff you bring home, however, you need to make white flour anathema. To quote *Seinfeld*'s George Costanza, anathema means, "They don't like it."

You need to learn to not like white flour.

Now I realize some baked goods aren't going to work with whole-wheat flour. For me, it's Yorkshire pudding. I have made them with whole-wheat flour *and they were just fine!* Not to hear my wife and kids tell it, though. I damn near had a rebellion on my hands. (Seriously, though, if you're baking a lot of stuff that requires white flour, you need to cut back on that.)

The big difference on the white flour front is going to be in the bread products you buy. When you cut white flour, you cut out a lot of garbage you might buy from the grocery store or other places. Many pastries and treats are white flour heavy, which means they're out most of the time. Cheese buns and many other kinds of buns are out too. And say goodbye to white flour bagels and white bread.

For bread, consider 100 percent whole-wheat whole-grain varieties that list this as the first ingredient: "Whole-grain whole-wheat flour including the germ." This is a good germ. Look for this. Buy this.

These breads have more fiber, less sugar, fewer other unpronounceable ingredients, are more filling, healthier, promote exercise performance better and are less likely to lead to overconsumption. Making this switch will retrain your taste buds so you come to dislike white flour. In the final step, when you cut fast food, it will be easier.

CUT Most Junk Food Snacks and REPLACE with Healthier Snacks

Ask the apple question. Instead of potato chips or candy, eat carrots and peas and apples and celery and grapes and strawberries and mini tomatoes and nuts and seeds . . . you get the idea.

Cut back on chips and chocolate and doughnuts and tarts and muffins and pastries and . . . you also get the idea.

You don't have to go all or nothing on this. I advise—at minimum—replacing 50 percent of your junk food snacks with healthier options. Consider shooting for 75 percent.

CUT Spreads/Sauces and REPLACE with *Less* Spreads/Sauces

I remember watching a relative butter his bread. I was blown away by the amount he used.

I love butter. I have it on toast every morning (along with eggs), but I'm spartan in my usage. I use just the barest amount to get coverage. Every time I use a spread of any type, or a sauce for that matter, I use just enough to get a good addition of flavor without going overboard.

It's a math game. Scoop out one *level* tablespoon of butter and see what it looks like. Memorize that size, and know that it contains 100 calories. How much do you need? You'll find you can get away with much less and that the reduction has an imperceptible effect on taste.

Any time you're adding a creamy sauce, mayo, cream cheese, a slice of cheese, another spread, etcetera, to food, think about the amount. Keep it as small as you can without making it seem that life sucks.

CUT Creamy Salad Dressings and REPLACE with Vinaigrettes

This is not as straightforward as it seems, as some vinaigrettes can be loaded with calories. You need to read labels and find ones that are low in calories. Also, just as with the spreads, don't use much. I have a powerful-tasting Greek vinaigrette I prefer and the amount I use on a large salad amounts to only 20 calories.

CUT Cereal and REPLACE with Eggs

I eat eggs for breakfast almost every day. Cereal—even the stuff you think might be good—is not good. It's packed with calories, it's heavily refined and it's not filling. A trick manufacturers employ is to use multiple types of sugar so they don't have to list "sugar" as the first ingredient. Read the ingredient "fine print" and watch for brown sugar, corn syrup, high-fructose corn syrup, fructose and molasses. Taken all together, these "stealth" sugars can make sugar the leading ingredient. Not surprisingly, cutting cereal further lowers your sweetness threshold.

By comparison, eggs have only 70 calories each, taste awesome, are unprocessed and healthy, and have a high satiety factor.

Cereal is quick and convenient, but it takes no time to get good at cooking eggs fast. Getting up five minutes earlier won't kill you. Have eggs for breakfast.

CUT *Most* Restaurant Meals and REPLACE with Home-cooked Meals/Packed Lunches

It's the sit-down restaurant meals I'm talking about here. We're not cutting fast food until the final step. Allow me to explain why.

Restaurant meals are more dangerous than fast food meals for a few reasons:

- They taste better
- The portions are larger
- There is more choice
- There is the bread basket
- There are appetizers
- There is dessert
- There are doggie bags
- There are buffets

A lot of people can't handle too many fast food meals. They just get gross after a while. But if there were some kind of *Star Trek* transporter diet plan that "beamed" the extra unhealthy calories from restaurant food out of my stomach after eating—and if I could afford it—I could eat every meal at good restaurants every single day. There is so much choice and it often all tastes so good.

Read *The End of Overeating* and you'll know why it tastes so good. The chicken breasts I make don't taste half as good as the ones I can get in a restaurant, and there's a reason for that: I don't impregnate them with a ton of fat, sugar and salt that causes them to melt in my mouth and adds a ton more calories. Restaurant food can seem unprocessed yet still be processed to hell and back. The addition of fat means chewing is minimal because it makes food softer, so you can eat faster and take in more calories.[2] Even seemingly healthy vegetables are often deep-fried in oil to make them taste better, adding a load of extra calories.

Another example: When I make mashed potatoes, I use milk and a little butter. Restaurants often use whipped cream and lots of butter. All these extra calories add up fast.

You need to make restaurant meals for special occasions. It's rare that I go out for dinner. And when I do, the kids are usually left behind. My wife and I save those outings for date nights and we savor them. Because I rarely eat at a restaurant, when I do, I get to go berserk. I order *whatever the hell I want*. Because it's a rare treat, I throw caloric awareness to the wind and pig out big time. I've earned it.

Earn it. Make it rare, and make it special.

Remember that we have free recipes for healthy, lower-calorie meals on my website, www.BodyForWife.com. Also, a registered dietitian can be a valuable resource to take you around the grocery store and show you how to shop if you're unsure of what to do.

If you travel a great deal and *must* eat at restaurants all the time, or if regular business lunches are a requirement, you need to find a way to restrain calories while eating out. One resource you can check out is the book *The Portion Teller*, by Lisa Young.

CUT Mindlessly Reaching for Food and REPLACE with Stopping and Thinking

Exercise has strengthened your brain to make better decisions by now, so use that power. Decide if the pleasure is worth the calories. Think about whether you want it. Determine how much you'll have and if you'll be able to stop after a reasonable amount. Often, stopping and thinking will make you realize that you're not so much hungry as bored, or frustrated, or angry. If you're truly hungry, and do want whatever you're reaching for, go for it. At least you're eating mindfully.

CUT Alcohol Intake by Another 25 Percent and REPLACE with Water

Again, no explanation required.

And now I'll remind you that *it's okay* to hold fast here. This is it for Level 2, and while it certainly involves effort to get to this point, you'll find with practice that it's sustainable without making you feel you've sold yourself into weight loss slavery. I made it to Level 2, more or less, and stayed there *for 10 years* before I moved on to Level 3. I'd lost 30 pounds and looked good and was healthy. When I was ready to up my game, see my abs and get super fit, I took it to another level.

If you complete both parts of Level 2 and hold firm, you're doing great. You're doing way better than the majority of people on the planet. Be proud.

And when you're ready—when you want to—go to Level 3. Become a Workout Warrior. That, in turn, will make you want to pursue the dietary changes: Eating for Excellence.

12

THE VIRTUOUS CYCLE, LEVEL 3

When you stop doing things for fun you might as well be dead.

—ERNEST HEMINGWAY

This evolution can take a decade.

If this thought scares you, tell me what other all-important plans you have for the next 10 years.

It's progression versus stagnation, or even regression. Say you're 40. Ten years from now you could be much fitter, carrying around a lot less fat and much more muscle, be running marathons or climbing mountains, hoisting kettlebells or kayaking oceans, cycling the countryside or swimming the sea, looking and feeling great, excited about the next 50 years of your life and unable to imagine the person you used to be.

Or you could just be 10 years closer to death.

There is nothing wrong with the micro-pace; your body *and* mind need time to adjust. If you've been overweight and inactive and eating junk for a long time, you'll experience a psychological and physiological rebellion at changing all that. Just know that time is on your side. Jack LaLanne always said it was never too late to start, and he was right.

Level 3 isn't for everyone, but you can give it a shot. How do you know if you're ready to go for it? Well, if living at Level 2 has become comfortable, this is a good indication. If you feel you're ready for a new challenge, if vanity is calling to you even more and you want to be a little slimmer or a little more muscular. If you want to run a longer race, faster. If you want to be even stronger, kick even more ass . . .

If you read this section and say, "Yeah, I want that," you're ready for Level 3.

LEVEL 3, EXERCISE: WORKOUT WARRIOR

A Workout Warrior, in my book, is someone who goes hard a good six hours a week or more. This is where ambitious fitness, health and weight loss goals are achieved. This is where you start to get amazing visual outcomes and major improvements in physical performance. It's not mandatory that you become a full-blown Workout Warrior, but this is where life starts to get rock star, so don't rule it out as a possibility.

I am a Workout Warrior and my body is a great place to live. Oh, and you know how I've harped on about caloric burn not being that significant a contributor to weight loss? That's not always true for Workout Warriors. We can burn a lot of calories each week; it adds up.

"I've been consciously physically active for 20 years, but more so in the last 10 because I eat like a horse and I don't want to weigh 300 pounds," singer Sarah McLachlan told me. She explained her diet to me and she's exaggerating about the horse part, but Sarah does enjoy her French fries. She also has an intense fitness regimen, which, while not a license to run amok dietarily, does provide caloric leeway. But of course her motivations go far beyond being able to eat more.

"I also really like the way I feel when I exercise," she said. "It energizes me and is a great stress reliever."

For me, a slow week is six hours of exercise. Six *hard* hours. Not only have I made my body used to this, but I've also taught it to crave such intense efforts. Sometimes I average closer to eight or even 10 hours, especially in the summer when my bike and I are good friends.

I have a wife, kids and a lot of demands on my time, but fitness is my number one hobby. This is my playtime. I don't watch double-header football games or putter around in the garage or play *World of Warcraft* or watch too much TV. It's okay to like these things, but exercise needs to be high on your priority list.

Margaret is also a busy person. And she runs like the wind. A lot.

I've learned to love exercise so much that if I won the lottery and didn't have to work, I'd spend even more time working out. When you achieve Workout Warrior status, you start trying to jig your schedule to find more time to exercise. You seem to be on a continual mission to increase your **FILD.**

We Workout Warriors are a little crazy that way. You can be that way too. You'd be welcome in our asylum. It's fun here.

"Gym was what I thought about all day," Kyle Shewfelt, an Olympic gymnast who took gold in Athens 2004, told me. "It was just so much fun being upside down and figuring out what crazy things my body could do."

"My passion for the sport and people who enjoy propelling themselves through a winter landscape along with me is something I tap into even in my racing," Olympic cross-country skier Chandra Crawford told me. "On the sunny day in Italy when I woke up to my chance to race the world's best, what did I focus on? To live the day with full undiluted passion for the sport. It worked!"

It sure did. Crawford won gold in Torino 2006.

This mentality takes a long time to develop. Virtuous Cycle scheduling aside, you may need to spend years in the Fitness Focused level to achieve it. Be patient and persevere. If you want it to, it will come.

What will come? Well, as with Level 2, there will be a focus on added frequency of exercise, increased intensity, lengthier training sessions and further experimentation with other types of activity that are more difficult (remember, it's all about getting FILD). But the difference this time is that you'll be looking for these things because you want them, you crave them, not because we're telling you this is what you need to do.

Believe it or not, this level is less about pushing your body than it is about pushing your brain. Train your mind to crave it, and the body just gets pushed. Not only that, but this improved mental toughness further improves your ability to make better food choices. Don't forget that part.

Positive Self-talk

It's not just general attitudes that matter but also situational ones that take place from moment to moment during exercise.

Remember the story *The Little Engine That Could*? He/she/it was going up that hill and saying, "I think I can, I think I can," over and over. This is positive self-talk. It's about using a bit of self-hypnosis to hype yourself up and focus on the task at hand. Professional athletes use it all the time.

Imagine this scenario: You are an offensive lineman in the NFL and some 300-pound monstrosity across from you wants to mow you down so he can rip your quarterback's spleen out. Knowing your quarterback can't throw touchdowns without his spleen, you want to do a good job and prevent this defender getting past. You can't be thinking, *This guy is going to kill me*. Instead, you have to believe this: *I'm going to mess him up. I'm going to hit him so hard that his grandchildren will be born dizzy.*

Now that's a winning attitude.

I know you don't play in the NFL, and you probably don't get into too many situations where people's spleens are at stake, but there is merit in having a "No prisoners!" approach to exercise. Here are some examples that might be more applicable to your life:

Lifting weights:
- *Bad*: I feel weak. My lifting is going to be awful today. I don't even know why I bothered coming to the gym.
- *Good*: I feel as if I've got a mini Schwarzenegger in each butt cheek. I'm going to do some serious squats today!

Planning a run after work:
- *Bad*: This day was a major drag. It could teach things that suck how to suck. I don't want to run today. I want ice cream washed down with gin and tonic.
- *Good*: I can't wait to get out of this office and go for a run outside. It's going to be awesome!

Coming up to a hill on your bicycle:
- *Bad*: I hate this hill. I'm going to walk my bike up it.
- *Good*: I'm going to make this hill beg for mercy.

Adopting a new fitness program:
- *Bad*: Another year, another broken New Year's resolution.
- *Good*: I'm excited about learning this new exercise. It's going to be fun.

I'm more in favor of motivating people with scientific facts rather than inspirational quotations, but there is one that comes to mind that seems appropriate. It was said by Henry Ford: "If you think you can do a thing, or think you can't do a thing, you are right."

Final Thoughts on Exercise

I know we've rammed a lot of science down your throat in this book, but to wrap up my final thoughts on exercise I'm going to channel Oprah just a little. Are you ready for the group hug?

I want you to think about what it means for you to be a Workout Warrior. What is it like for *you* to push yourself to the wall?

Now imagine that you've been exercising for a while, and you're Fitness Focused. You've been training pretty hard, making physical improvements, and now it's time to take it to the next, butt-kicking level.

But perhaps you're a little afraid—you maybe got that way when I started throwing around those "six-plus hours a week" numbers—because this is where things get real. This is where you find out what you're made of. Just FYI, finding out what you're made of is painful.

And awesome. Don't forget awesome.

Now let's do one of those visualization exercises. I want you to think about the next time you're exercising. It could be running, cycling, weightlifting, in a boot camp, in a pool or even in your extreme yoga class. Think about what it would be like to push it as hard as you can and keep it there. Think about the pain, then think about embracing it. Imagine your lungs rasping and your legs burning and your sweat pouring. Imagine that it's a while until it's over and you still push until the end.

Now imagine how it feels when it stops.

Well, you usually think *Thank God that's over* for a while, but imagine what it's like *after* you no longer feel as if you might blow your groceries and pray for death or pass out (note: hyperbole). I mean, think hard about it. Consider what it feels like inside your mind to find out how far and how hard you can physically push yourself. Wonder what it's like to *revel* in the fact that *today, I went as hard as I could*.

Do you think it's going to feel good? Well, you'd be wrong. It feels much better than good.

Do you want that feeling? Are you ready for that feeling? If yes, you're ready to become a Workout Warrior, so go out there and push it to the wall.

And then push through.

LEVEL 3, EATING: EATING FOR EXCELLENCE

Are we there yet?

Yes, we're there. Well, except for the troubleshooting chapter and the conclusion. That stuff is important too. Make sure you read it.

But first, let's finish this.

CUT Fast Food and REPLACE with Home-cooked Meals

I'm not saying you have to cut all fast food, but you're at a point now that it can become a lot more rare. You've worked with your schedule. You're figuring things out. You've got the slow cooker and the Glass Lock container thing happening to make sure you've always got healthy meals to choose in case of emergency, meals that can go from freezer to nuker and be ready in minutes.

You're better at planning for thawing things out, making food on the fly with fresh ingredients, or just settling for grilled cheese sandwiches and a bowl of grapes or some sliced up oranges. Dinner at home doesn't always have to be some big time-sucking event. Fast food is for emergencies, for those situations when you have no choice because time ran away from you. It happens to everyone, but work on making it happen less often.

CUT Eating until Full and REPLACE with Eating until Satisfied

In chapter 6, I mentioned an old Chinese adage, "Eat until you are eight-tenths full." You don't have to clean your plate. You don't have to be stuffed. You can experiment and learn how much food you need to make it to your next meal without being ravenous. The trick is to be *fueled*. Never starving, never stuffed. And only a little hungry before bed.

For the emotional eaters—those eating for psychological rather than physiological reasons—exercise should by now have made a serious dent in this problem, as explained in chapter 4. So use the new willpower to your advantage. And in the spur of the moment, if you feel a desire to binge, consider a brief exercise binge instead until the feeling passes.

CUT Frozen/Boxed Dinners and REPLACE with Fresh Ingredients

Eating at home isn't such a great thing if what you're eating is chicken strips, fish sticks and salt-laden dinners out of a box. That stuff is garbage. You need to cut that out and get a bit of your chef on. As I said, it doesn't always have to be fancy. Know that you'll learn how to be efficient and throw something together last minute that's fresh, lower in calories and healthy. You'll learn how to shop in a way that ensures you always have these ingredients on hand. It takes some time to develop this kind of skill power. Keep working on it, and remember the free recipes on my site.

CUT Back Fatty Meats and REPLACE with Leaner Choices

In chapters 2 and 5, we talked about the dangers of fat. If you need a refresher, suffice it to say that fatty foods have a high caloric density and are extra yummy, a fact that promotes overconsumption. By cutting back on fatty meats, you can lower both calories and reward value, the latter of which further serves to lower caloric intake because you eat less.

Most red meat is higher in fat, though cuts such as flank and top sirloin steak, as well as extra-lean ground beef, are better choices. Poultry without the skin is lean, but if the skin is on, it's a fatty choice. Bacon is fatty too, which is why it tastes so awesome. Some fish is fatty, like salmon, but these are mostly healthy fats, so they're okay.

So choose the leaner cuts of meat and remove the skin from chicken.

CUT Back on Red Meat and REPLACE with Poultry and Fish

This is an additional way to reduce calories, because chicken and fish can be more satiating for a lower number of calories, as long as they're not battered and/or deep-fried. Part of the reason is that many people perceive red meat to have a higher reward value. They like it more, so it's easier to eat more.

Another reason for making this switch is to improve health.

See, red meat, especially the smoked/packaged varieties such as bacon, sausage, baloney and ham, can be seriously unhealthy. A number of studies show that they cause a profound increase in both cardiovascular disease and cancer.[1] Another interesting study, which appeared in the *Annals of Internal Medicine* in 2010, looked at 12,555 deaths over a 26-year period. It showed that people who ate plant-based low-carbohydrate diets were fine, but "a low-carbohydrate diet based on animal sources was associated with higher all-cause mortality in both men and women."[2]

Fatty fish such as salmon, mackerel and tuna is great for you, and easy to prepare. My grocery store often has salmon on for cheap because the next day is the best-before date, and I have an excellent money-saving strategy. I buy a bunch and freeze some, plus cook some that night. Salmon that's getting close to its best-before can taste a little fishier, but a few drops here and there of lemon juice prior to cooking make that disappear. It tastes fresh. My family can never tell the difference.

CUT Back on Meat for Dinner and REPLACE with Vegetarian Dinner

Try it now and then. Start with once a week. Get the family involved. It won't kill you.

CUT Eating before Bed and REPLACE with . . . Nothing

Well, not *nothing*. Remember the strategies we gave you in chapter 6 for going to bed a little hungry? Try those instead of eating.

Going to bed a little hungry is one of the most effective weight loss strategies that I know. You focus on staying fueled throughout the day. Eat breakfast, eat lunch, have a small second lunch or a light snack, eat dinner and then *stop!*

It's a tough one to do at first, but try. You don't have to do it every night, but if you're determined, this is one you can get good at, and it becomes sustainable.

Crash diets aren't sustainable because the intense hunger causes pain, and in this land of plenty you can only put up with such suffering for so long before you lose your mind and inhale half the menu at the Cheesecake Factory. The beauty of going to bed hungry is that the pain is much less and the time period is short, because appetite largely resets overnight.

You will be hungry when you wake up, making you want to eat breakfast, and that's a good thing.

Just remember not to go to bed so hungry that you get up and eat in the middle of the night.

Final Tip—the Booze

If you can cut a bit more alcohol too, do that. Or not. Your call.

Okay, grasshopper, we've come a long way. It's time to wrap this book up. Next is a troubleshooting chapter about dealing with illness and injury, and then we're on to my final words on how you can keep this amazing new body of yours.

Turn the page . . .

13

TROUBLESHOOTING: DEALING WITH INJURIES AND ILLNESS

If you're going through hell, keep going.

—WINSTON CHURCHILL

And now we enter the "If I can do it, so can you" portion of the book.

Sometimes the body gets hurt or sick, and it needs rest. But sometimes people rest too much. They allow an injury or a chronic condition to stop them from living a full life, not understanding that pushing through discomfort to force a body to improve can actually force a body to improve. This doesn't mean do something stupid, but most problems don't get fixed while you're horizontal.

I realize that inspirational stories aren't a scientifically supported method of behavior change. The examples throughout this book provide context and anecdotal support for the science-based thesis we present. If inspirational stories alone could do the job, those who read the *Chicken Soup for the Soul* books would be the happiest, most successful and well-adjusted people on the planet. (I suppose I should mention I had two exercise-type stories published in those chicken soup books. Don't hate.)

Anyway, it's simple: you don't fix your body lying in bed. I mean, if you have the flu and feel as if you've been hit by a truck, you need rest. And please don't tell me about the color of your snot. But even if you have some lifelong debilitating condition, continual bed rest = downhill slide.

There's good evidence to show that regular exercise and other healthy habits can improve your immunity, but it goes beyond that. One of exercise's best contributions to dealing not just with illness but with injury is that it makes you stronger. If you're weak, any kind of condition is going to kick your ass harder than if you're strong. When you build a strong suit of armor down to your literal core, you can shrug off a host of maladies with much greater ease than if you're a weak, sedentary blob.

There's also the physical therapy aspect. If you're broken, you need to make your body fix itself. I have much personal experience with this. And yes, I'm going to tell you about it.

Here are some stories of people who told me how exercise helped them recover from illness and injury. Plus there's the one from me. Yes, I talk to myself.

Perhaps you can take motivation from learning about real people conquering physical adversity with physical fitness.

MONTEL WILLIAMS: FIGHTING A DELAYING ACTION AGAINST MULTIPLE SCLEROSIS

Emmy-winner Montel Williams is not your typical pot-smoking snowboarder.

In 1999 Williams was diagnosed with multiple sclerosis, and it hit him hard. After a downward slide to rock bottom, Williams decided to get his life back.

"The doctor said I'd be in a wheelchair in four years, and I just wanted to quit," Williams told me. "I almost took my own life; the depression lasted about seven months. But now I'm looking to live instead of looking to die."

At a certain point, Montel felt the need to go against doctor's orders.

"Despite what the doctor said, I should have continued working out with weights," he said. "I abruptly stopped doing that on his recommendation, and from 2000 to 2006 I wasn't training that hard. It was much more calisthenic. I finally realized I needed to start pushing the muscles.

From 2006, I've been learning more and more from physiologists at Canyon Ranch in Arizona to deal with the loss of muscle mass."

And he's staying out of the wheelchair. Williams also credits exercise, a diet high in raw vegetables and his participation in an experimental treatment out of the University of Wisconsin that electrically stimulates the brain via the tongue to help it create new neural pathways.

This determination—and the results it garnered—allowed him to return to a sport he loves. Soon after we spoke he was off to go helicopter snowboarding in Alaska.

And the pot? That's not while on the slopes. Montel is a champion of its medical use; he found it to be of great benefit for mitigating lower-extremity pain and reducing leg spasticity while sleeping.

KRIS McPARLAND: THROWING LUPUS FOR A LOOP

Kris McParland, 45, is a corporate manager and mother of two in Nanaimo, British Columbia. We went to high school together. She is very pretty.

In 2008, she was diagnosed with lupus, a systemic autoimmune disease.

"The challenge for me was overwhelming fatigue and pain," she told me. "I wasn't on any treatment, just pain control. I wasn't able to walk because of the arthritis in my feet. I went through a three-month process of just trying to get out of bed, and I had to take a sick leave from my career."

Faced with life in a wheelchair, she found a good rheumatologist who put her on the right medication, which kick-started her return to mobility. "I was able to get physical again, but you go through cycles of flare-remission and it becomes very easy to take a day off and it snowballs quickly. I had to make a deal with myself that I have to work out even on bad days. I realize that the first five minutes are going to be hell, but then you break through that and kick in the reward system." She says this reward from exercise is far greater than any reward from sitting on the couch and watching TV.

"Exercise is absolutely making the remissions longer, the flare-ups less intense. It's helping to hold my lupus at bay. I feel better if I move."

She was doing aerobic workouts, then started with a trainer to push her with weightlifting to strengthen her body. "This has made the lupus better to the point where I've been able to cut my medication in half. It's been better for not just my body but my spirit as well. I'm back to where I was pre-diagnosis."

TONY SEKULLICH: SWEATING AWAY THE DIABETES

In 2012, I wrote an article for my *Chicago Tribune* column about using exercise to combat type 2 diabetes. Dr. Michael Joyner of the Mayo Clinic and Dr. Tim Church of the Pennington Biomedical Research Center both told me the same thing: exercise is by far the most important factor in reversing this disease. Take your meds and cut back on sugar, but you must exercise.

And that's what Tony Sekullich, a 42-year-old television writer in Toronto, did. In 2011 he was feeling like a dog's breakfast. He was lethargic, had a rapid heartbeat and couldn't concentrate on his work. He went to the doctor and after blood work learned that his fasting blood glucose level was 310 mg/dL. This was way beyond the normal range of 72–108 mg/dL.

Like Church and Joyner, Tony's doctor told him exercise was the critical component, and Sekullich took it to heart.

"I was so out of shape that at first I would go for only five-mile bike rides," he said. His diet changed too, but not dramatically. He replaced soda with water, ate more fruit and ate less. He also started taking the drug Metformin.

"After a few weeks, I built up stamina on my bike and added in some swimming too," said Sekullich. With the dietary changes and drug therapy, his fasting glucose had dropped a month later to 155 mg/dL, and the target for most patients with diabetes is below 126 mg/dL, so getting better. "My doctor was surprised I'd turned it around so fast."

Sekullich kept up with the lifestyle change, adding more exercise—including starting a weightlifting regimen—and losing close to 20 pounds. After another four months his fasting glucose had dropped to 108 mg/dL—within the target range—and his Metformin dosage was cut in half. Six months later Tony saw his doctor again. "He said I now have it totally under control and he's taking me off the Metformin completely and wants me to keep on top of it with diet and exercise alone."

LYNN LEROUX: FIGHTING FIBROMYALGIA

Fifty-three-year-old Lynn Leroux—one of my clients—was diagnosed with fibromyalgia in the early 1990s; she had been experiencing pain for 30 years. "I was getting extremely fatigued and couldn't even do something simple like empty the dishwasher," she told me. "I was just so tired all the time.

"My husband [whom I know to be a fan of fitness—he's the one who inspired me to quest for completing an Ironman triathlon] always pushed me to my limit," she said. "The early years were really tough and I just had to push through it." But she kept pushing, because she wanted to be able to go cycling with her husband and keep up.

At least that was her goal in the early years. "But now I push myself," she told me.

More recently Lynn has taken up weightlifting. "It's made a huge difference because it's given me a lot of strength," she said. "Now that I have some core strength I can do so much more than I could before. I'm in a much better place now. The pain is still there, but I can do more and for much longer and more frequently because I'm stronger."

Lynn experiences much less fatigue now that she's started weightlifting, and she credits a weight loss goal for her most recent accomplishments. "It wasn't just about fibromyalgia anymore," Lynn told me. "There were definitely some vanity goals that helped as well. I didn't like being overweight and I've lost 20 pounds and am only five pounds away from my goal."

JANE SEYMOUR: PILATES LETS HER PLAY

"I came to Hollywood in 1976 and discovered Pilates," actor Jane Seymour told me. "At that time there would be about five people in the studio. It was Kate, Jackie and Farrah—the Charlie's Angels—and Joan Collins and myself. We all knew each other. It was pretty amazing. That was before anyone knew about Pilates."

And after she'd had surgery on her lower back for bulging disks, it was Pilates that returned her to health.

"Pilates is perfect for anyone who has had an injury," Seymour said. "They use it for injured dancers. It's about body alignment, core strength and flexibility. It's an amazing workout." She explained that she uses what's called a Gyrotonic machine, "which has pulleys and straps, and it's almost like you're churning milk. It's fantastic for rotation of the spine . . . I absolutely credit this machine and Jeeny [Seymour's Pilates instructor] to helping support my back. I work very hard on my core strength; it's important for my body." And it's allowed her to stay active.

"I love to play golf, although it's not necessarily a good movement with my back issues, but Pilates allows me to play." And not just golf but rediscovering lost passions. Before becoming an actor, Seymour danced with the Kirov ballet company. "One of the great joys in my life was doing *Dancing with the Stars*. It was the hardest thing I've ever done as well as one of the most fun and exciting. Dancing with a bad back at my age—and having to do it live—was huge. I loved learning that it was something I could still do. It brought back something into my life and made me realize how much I missed it."

MARTY SCOTT: THE 320-POUND RUNNER

By itself, being over 300 pounds is neither an illness nor an injury, but it can prevent you from engaging in certain activities. Or can it?

Many say they're too overweight to run, but that didn't stop 42-year-old Marty Scott, a city planner and father of two in Chicago.

"I started out with just walking," he told me. "The big issue was making time for it." See? NOT his weight but TIME! He had a good attitude about his physical capabilities from the start.

"I would integrate short runs into these walks, and they got longer and longer. Then some friends suggested I do a 5K Thanksgiving Day race and it was a lot of fun and very motivating."

Then he did a 10K race in 80 minutes, which isn't so fast, but it's much faster than a walking pace. Now he can run a 10K race in an hour, and that *is* running.

And he's going farther too. Scott is up to eight-mile races. *Eight-mile runs weighing 320 pounds*. And now he's working on the diet side to get his weight down. Running has been a life-changing catalyst for him.

ME: I BLAME THE MORPHINE

I've had low-back issues since high school. I'm pretty sure they started with me trying to show off how much I could deadlift in 10th-grade gym class while having no clue as to proper technique. I had flare-ups and issues on and off for years, until 2003, when things really blew up.

I'd been working out for a decade at that point, and had to suffer through back pain during exercise. But in September 2003 I'd had a terrible cough that would not die. The constant hacking put my low back in further jeopardy, and when I bent over to hoist a full laundry basket from the floor, I broke into another coughing fit, and my lower lumbar exploded. I collapsed to the floor and cried like a kid who's had his Halloween candy stolen.

I could not walk. Tylenol 3 did nothing. After four days of continuous downhill slide, I was taken to the emergency room in a wheelchair. The first thing they did was give me a load of IV morphine, which took the edge off. I still screamed when they moved me from gurney to CT scanner, though.

The scan showed two bulging disks low in my lumbar vertebrae. Surgery was mentioned and I blurted out, "No [expletive] surgery!"

The doctor said I'd be in for a long rehab, which I said I could do. "Oh, and you can forget about any more weightlifting," he said.

"Go [expletive] yourself," I replied. I blame the morphine. Usually I'm nice to doctors, being married to one and all.

I went through a pile of Percocet over the next couple of weeks while regaining the ability to walk, then weaned down to Tylenol 3 while meeting with the physiotherapist for the Calgary Flames. Long story short, it was three months of mind-numbing torture. I needed the therapist for only three sessions to show me what to do, and then I spent that quarter of the year doing back rehabilitation and core-strengthening work to return to normal. By the time 2004 arrived, it was as if the blowout had never happened. In fact, my back was stronger than I could ever remember.

Now I can ski through moguls and off cliffs with reckless abandon. Now I can jump over fences or run down treacherous trails at high speeds. Now I can ride my road bike hunched over for hours. Now I can lift heavy weights without putting my back in jeopardy, no matter what that doctor said.

Sometimes you just need to err on the side of "go for it."

CRAIG McARTHUR AND CHRIS FROLEK: THE KNEED FOR SPEED

Oh, man, I suck at puns.

Craig McArthur is my best friend. If I'm at a Rush concert, he's there with me. And when we're skiing the expert runs and stop to look over a perilous cliff and I say to him, "You first," he goes first.

Did I mention that Craig has had six surgeries on his knee?

Dr. Mark Heard, the consulting physician for the Canadian Alpine Ski Team and Canadian Freestyle Ski Team, told me that the success rate for knee surgery "is in the 95 percent area" for all patients, from elite athletes to amateurs. "They generally return to the same level or higher after recovering from their reconstruction," he said.

And yet many see it as a death knell for athleticism. But not Chris Frolek, a 35-year-old registered nurse in Calgary who was playing competitive tennis when he tore his ACL in a doubles match in 2008.

Like many facing a long rehab from an anterior cruciate ligament injury, Chris found that being off his game had a depressing effect. "I was feeling very down, but I did everything they told me to do," he said. "Staying active by doing the stretching and exercises they gave me, along with lots of time on a stationary bike, had a positive effect on my mood."

And he's keeping his spirits up with ambitious recovery goals. "I want to get into the top 100 tennis players in Canada," he told me. "I was on my way before the injury, and it's a goal I haven't given up on." He also intends to do a full Ironman triathlon before he turns 50. Completing a 2.4-mile swim and a 112-mile bike race and running a full marathon is not the ambition of a man who intends to let knee surgery slow him down.

LIZ CLAMAN: THE EMMY WINNER WITH A TWISTED SPINE

Liz Claman is an Emmy-winning anchor for Fox Business Network. She is also a marathoner and triathlete with scoliosis. A specialist said she'd never be an athlete and that running was out of the question.

Claman told me she obeyed the rules and didn't do much for exercise throughout her life, "until I decided to break the rules. I wanted to be an athlete." For her, wanting to become an athlete changed everything else.

"I was 38 and professionally feeling like I was in a rut, and I was too tired to change it," she told me. "So I decided to work on the physical part instead. I decided that I could run the New York marathon to crack the shell that had grown around me," she said. "I approached a trainer at my gym who completely inspired me. He said I could do anything I wanted, and we put a plan together."

Claman said her hips always hurt on her runs, and she and her trainer came up with some stretches to compensate, but at the beginning of the New York marathon in 2005, she said, "I could feel pain in my hip after the first step, and I started to panic." But she still finished the race, and she ran the whole way, with no stopping to walk.

"In every part of my life I was able to break those rules. Professionally my career has soared and I have to believe there is a connection. I have to wonder whether I'd have been able to advance professionally if I hadn't broken through the physical barriers first."

FEEL FREE TO QUOTE ME

I wrote an article about overcoming illness and injury for AOL long ago. A couple of years later a woman wrote to tell me about how one sentence in that article changed her life. She was able to fight against debilitating rheumatoid arthritis to reduce her pain, increase her energy levels and enjoy life a lot more by taking up exercising.

She quoted the article's sentence in her email: "If you don't conquer your illnesses and injuries, you allow them to conquer you."

It isn't Shakespeare, but it's true. You may not cure yourself, but you can better your situation. You can make a stronger, healthier body that can deal with physical travails far easier.

You can conquer rather than be conquered.

CONCLUSION:

LONG-TERM SUSTAINABILITY

Always dream and shoot higher than you know you can do.
Do not bother just to be better than your contemporaries or
predecessors. Try to be better than yourself.

—WILLIAM FAULKNER

I am not yet in the best shape of my life.

I have a bucket list, an exercise bucket list. Also, I have a desire to look better. I can see about four abs, but I'm always questing for more. Unfortunately, six-packs of beer and six-pack abs are mutually exclusive.

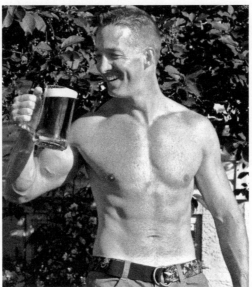

Shown: Ab filler.

Life has become a series of physical quests for me. Recall the theory of planned behavior from chapter 7? It's the one that says having a positive attitude and planning for future accomplishments increases the likelihood of adhering to a new behavior.

I don't have to worry about going back to the way I was, because I'm always trying to get in better shape. True, one day I will peak, and then all my efforts will be put into a valiant delaying action against age, but that day has not yet come. I am currently training to qualify for the Boston Marathon, and one day I'd like to complete an Ironman triathlon, go helicopter skiing, run a 10K in under 40 minutes and surf a big wave.

Well, maybe not too big a wave.

This thinking needs to become your way too. You need to continuously strive to get better, not because you have to but because you *want* to. Because you've learned to feel the love of your chosen activities. Because the exercise you do has come to define you as a person. Because you've embraced your competitive spirit. Because you want to *carpe* more *diems*.

When you finish one race, book the next. Think of things you can do that require you to go farther, get faster, be stronger. Pick a race that requires more toughness or is a longer distance. Decide there's a fitness class that won't be out of your league for long. Try a new exercise that looks hard and strive to be good at it. Pick a cycling loop that you have to train hard to complete. Learn to walk fast and far enough that you tire the dog out instead of the other way around. Run a marathon, or walk one. Be determined to hold those challenging yoga poses. Swim an extra length. Put some more weight on the barbell . . .

Do all this, fuel it with good food, and you won't worry about gaining the weight back.

Life can be stagnation. Life can be a grind. Life can be filled with pain and sickness and sadness.

Or life can be adventure.

It was Helen Keller who said, "Life is either daring adventure or nothing at all."

I am not yet in the best shape of my life, and neither are you. Just because you can't do something today doesn't mean you can't do it one day.

It's time to start planning your next adventure. It's time to seize the day.

Seize it. And kick its ass.

ACKNOWLEDGEMENTS

I'm not sure how I'm supposed to do this.

Writers thanking editors isn't a cliché. Editors are awesome and deserve our thanks. They make us better because they love our work. I've never seen someone write in the acknowledgements, "My editor sucked. All we did was fight."

My editor did not suck. Linda Pruessen was amazing to work with. Sure, writers often thank their "amazing editor," but mine really is. Amazing, I mean. The draft I handed in and the version in your hands are way different. Because of Linda, you got to read something a lot better.

I also owe Michelle MacAleese a sincere thank you for championing this book at Random House Canada. She helped make it happen. Pamela Murray was wonderful working through all the final stages and details, and I also want to thank Alison Reid for her careful copyediting (and for saying such nice things about the book).

And there are also the terrific editors who helped me get here over hundreds of articles. Sam, who I think deserves the title of "discovering" me; and Rosie, who listened when I cold-called the *LA Times*, and can almost pretend to like Rush. I also need to thank Jen for helping me figure out the broader picture, and Mary for always sounding happy to get a call from me, and Karen for saying I make her laugh. I also loved working with Robyn and Tami and James and Elysha and Emma and Chris and Kim and Jay and others who ripped my work apart to make me better. Even though I've cursed you all from time to time, thanks.

I don't think agents need any thanks from writers at all. They get a percentage.

Ha—I'm just messing with you, David. You're awesome. You embraced the vision. Bike ride?

If I don't mention my wife soon, I'm going to be in deep poo. This is the "Well, duh!" portion of the acknowledgements. She made all this happen. I was much less a man before her. I may have written the words, but she did most of the work. I love her.

My kids screamed and beat the crap out of each other through much of the writing. I love them too.

Mom is on the list, of course. She was always my biggest fan. Kinda verged on stalking, actually. Love her as well. And everyone else I'm related to? You too. I don't want to single out dads (I have two) and sisters and cousins because if I do, someone will feel left out and then it's an angry email from an Australian uncle. If we share 1/64th DNA or better, I thank you. Happy now?

I have a feeling I suck at this.

Gotta do a shout-out to the best friend: Craig McArthur. I talk too much and only sometimes he tells me to shut up. He's put up with me talking about this book for years. Best ski partner ever.

Special thanks to my thesis adviser Professor Christon Archer, for telling me to "pick a hill and prepare to die on it." Also thanks to Hugo-winner Rob Sawyer for instructing me: "If you try to please everyone, you end up pleasing no one."

Steven Brust: Thirty years ago your Vlad Taltos character put a voice in my head that became a core of my desire to become a writer.

John Varley: You're damn funny. And eloquent. I learned from you.

Dr. Yoni Freedhoff: You always took time, and helped evolve my thinking on some important stuff about weight loss and just basic human decency. I trust you and am happy we are friends.

Lindy Kennedy: Thanks for making sure we weren't full of crap. Your knowledge of nutrition is top-notch.

And Dear Margaret:

How the hell did you ever put up with me?

You're a genius. My wife is the smartest person I ever met. Then one day she said, "I think Margaret is smarter than me." I didn't disagree. I'm going to say it's a close thing, though. You're both super geniuses. I need to make sure I'm clear on that. Both.

By the way, the kids want to borrow your dog again.

APPENDIX A:

SUPPLEMENTS AND PHARMACEUTICALS

If you've tried everything on the exercise and healthy eating front and success still eludes you, there are other options. And there's some good news about these options.

After a sordid history, a fairly safe and effective weight loss pharmaceutical is finally available. But it is a second-to-last resort. If you are a tough case, you may wish to discuss this with your physician.

QSYMIA (PHENTERMINE AND TOPIRAMATE)

Obesity expert Dr. Arya Sharma speaks highly of the possibilities for Qsymia, although he doesn't call it a weight loss drug. "The reason you turn to a medication is to prevent weight regain," he told me.

And that is the real issue. Many people do the yoyo weight loss. They can lose it, but they can't keep it off. "The pharmacology blocks the hunger response and can prevent metabolic slowdown," Sharma said.

He states that the drug is both effective and within tolerable safety parameters because it "is a combination of two drugs that have been around for decades and have been used by millions of people; we know exactly what the side effects are." He said most people tolerate it well because it's the unique combination of these drugs that makes them effective, and therefore allows for both of them to be at a low dose to minimize side effects.

What's more, "the testing on these drugs is far more extensive than testing for any weight loss drug ever before." But there can be side effects. This isn't a strategy to employ if you're looking to lean up for the beach; it should be used only if the risks associated with your current weight are higher than the risks of taking the medication. A doctor needs to make this call.

Dr. Yoni Freedhoff is more guarded. "The problem is that the physiology of appetite is so complex," he said. "You can get a drug to work on one pathway, but rest assured there are many others that will take up the slack." Evolution programmed these pathways to force us to eat. You know, so we don't die of starvation.

Again, it's a discussion to have with your physician.

WEIGHT LOSS SUPPLEMENTS

Unlike with pharmaceuticals, we DO make recommendations when it comes to weight loss supplements. Our recommendation is that they suck.

"The best supplements resulted in only two or three pounds of weight lost a year," Dr. Yoni Freedhoff told me.

A 2008 release from the US Food and Drug Administration sought to recall dozens of weight loss supplements because they were found to be contaminated with harmful substances. This is from the FDA release:

> "These tainted weight loss products pose a great risk to public health because they contain undeclared ingredients and, in some cases, contain prescription drugs in amounts that greatly exceed their maximum recommended dosages," said Janet Woodcock, M.D., director, Center for Drug Evaluation and Research, FDA. "Consumers have no way of knowing that these products contain powerful drugs that could cause serious health consequences."[1]

Bad, bad, bad. No, no, no.

APPENDIX B:

SURGICAL OPTIONS

For those who have truly reached their last resort with weight loss, this is the final option.

Society stigmatizes bariatric weight loss surgery as much as it stigmatizes the overweight, and that needs to stop. These procedures can make lives way better. In many cases, they *save lives*. Yes, bariatric surgery is often a lifesaving procedure that needs to be more available. People who scorn it are jerks.

Obesity expert Dr. Arya Sharma emphasizes that bariatric surgery is not a "cure" for being obese, and that substantial lifestyle changes are still required. What's more, success is measured in the alleviation of comorbidities (negative health consequences) rather than in pounds lost.

"The surgery has its risks," Dr. Sharma told me. "It's important to balance the risks of having it versus not having it. The more health problems you have, the better idea surgery appears to be."

And a 2009 analysis out of the Duke University Medical Center shows that the risk is less than previously believed. Dr. Eric DeMaria looked at almost 58,000 patients of bariatric surgery and found that the death rate from surgery was only 0.135 percent—a total of 78 people.

Complication rates were much higher, at 10 percent, with the most common complaint being nausea/vomiting. Over 200,000 people undergo bariatric surgery each year, making it one of the most common procedures performed in the United States.[1] Surgical techniques continue to advance to improve safety.

But it's important to note that this low mortality and complication rate data was accrued from participants in the Bariatric Surgery Centers of Excellence program. Not all surgeons qualify as excellent. *Caveat emptor.*

If you meet the criteria, if you've tried everything and feel that this is your last resort, do your homework and find a reputable clinic to discuss your surgical options. Yes, there are risks, but the benefits can be significant for those who have no other options. "With surgery, four out of five will be successful," Sharma said. It becomes a question of being in a desperate enough health situation to consider surgery as an option.

There are different types of surgery available, with the more challenging surgeries also being the more effective ones.

"The gold standard is the Roux-en-Y," Dr. Sharma said, referring to a form of gastric bypass. "It's more complex but has been around the longest and gets the best results." He explained that the sleeve gastrectomy is easier to do but less efficacious, and the adjustable gastric band (a lap band) is the easiest but leads to even less weight loss.

"I tell patients, 'If you want to make the surgeon's life easier, get a band. If you want to make your life easier, get a bypass,'" Sharma said.

I'm light-years from being an expert on this. Talk to more than one doctor.

APPENDIX C:

HEALTHY LIVING FOR YOUR CHILDREN

EXERCISE

All that stuff we wrote in chapter 4 about the benefits of exercise doesn't just apply to adults. Getting your children excited about physical activity can be one of the most important things you do as a parent. If you are concerned about your children's activity level, there is one thing you can do that will have a greater effect on their desire to exercise than anything else: *you must be a positive role model.*

"When children see you exercising, they mirror what you do," Dr. Teri McCambridge, director of sports medicine at Cincinnati Children's Hospital, told me. "If they see you get pleasure from it, they will as well." You need to put a positive spin on your exercise efforts for your children. Don't moan and groan about it. At least not in front of them.

Tips for Getting Kids Active

- Play together. Take them to the beach, kick a ball, go for walks, play catch or wrestle. Find creative ways to be active as a family.
- Remove pressure. If you go drill sergeant on them, they'll hate it. It's got to be encouraging and about having fun, because kids don't exercise, they play.
- Consider weightlifting. "Obese kids aren't going to be very good at aerobic activities," Dr. McCambridge, who also used to be head of the Council of Sport Medicine and Fitness for the American Academy of Pediatrics, told me. "Forcing them to engage in it

is hard on their joints and bad for their self-confidence." Weight training, on the other hand, often leads to a positive-feedback loop, according to Avery Faigenbaum, a pediatric exercise scientist and professor at the College of New Jersey in Ewing, NJ. "These kids are really strong," Faigenbaum told me. "The skinny kids are always impressed with how much the overweight kids can lift." Weightlifting will not stunt a child's growth. "We've done a 180-degree turn on this myth," he told me.

EATING

You are in charge. You are a parent first and a friend distant second. *You are in charge.*

"I don't hear from parents, 'My kids really like playing in traffic and I can't talk them out of it,'" Dr. David Katz said. "Letting your kids eat lots of junk food is like letting them play in traffic, only slower. Set the example, and don't take no for an answer."

But don't be an ogre. The kinder, gentler approach is the way to change your children's eating behaviors.

Tips for Improving Your Children's Eating Habits

- Again, be a good role model. In 2000, the *Journal of the American Dietetic Association* published a report revealing how five-year-old girls' ideas about dieting are influenced by their mothers' dieting habits. They found that women who dieted had young daughters who were twice as likely to know about dieting and to have developed ideas about it.[1] Throughout children's growth, parents' eating behaviors have a profound influence on the approaches their children take to food and diet. For girls this is especially problematic, because by the sixth grade 60 percent of them have been on a diet, and weight loss attempts can have an adverse effect on their physical and psychological health.[2]
- Engage them in the process. "You don't need to be a draconian policeman that always tells their kids what to eat," Dr. Yoni

Freedhoff said. "If they're old enough to talk about healthy eating, engage them in the process. Don't talk about body weight and bad foods versus good foods." Freedhoff likes the idea of having a family cooking night once a week—everyone gets involved and understands the ingredients being used and has a sense of ownership of the meal. It boosts confidence about their ability to eat healthily.

- Pick your battles. "But cultivate a world where there is less need for battle," Freedhoff said. Battles damage the parent–child relationship. You don't want to develop a fear of food in your child by saying things like, "You can't leave the table until you've cleaned your plate," or, "Eat your vegetables or you're having them for breakfast tomorrow."
- Be honest. Just talk to them. Make your children part of the healthy eating team. Get them to support *you* in your journey.

NOTES

INTRODUCTION

1. Keith Anderson, *Consumer Fraud in the United States, 2011: The Third FTC Survey*, March 2013, 20.
2. Michael Shermer, *Why People Believe Weird Things: Pseudoscience, Superstition, and Other Confusions of Our Time* (New York: St. Martin's Griffin, 2002), 275, 283–84.

1. WHY WE'RE FAT, PART I—THE WORLD WE LIVE IN

1. Katherine Flegel et al., "Prevalence and Trends in Obesity among U.S. Adults, 1999–2000," *Journal of the American Medical Association* 288, no. 14 (October 9, 2002): 1723–27.
2. Tim Church et al., "Trends over 5 Decades in U.S. Occupation-Related Physical Activity and Their Associations with Obesity," *PLoS ONE* 6, no. 5, epub (May 25, 2011).
3. Boyd Swinburn et al., "Increased Food Energy Supply Is More Than Sufficient to Explain the US Epidemic of Obesity," *American Journal of Clinical Nutrition* 90, no. 6 (September 2009): 1453–56.
4. Jeanine Stein, "Americans May Be Running Up the Calorie Count When Dining Out," *Los Angeles Times*, February 22, 2010.
5. Bruce Horovitz, "At Restaurants, Takeout Takes Off," *USA Today*, June 13, 2007.
6. Geoffrey James, "Stop Working More Than 40 Hours a Week," *Inc.*, April 24, 2012. http://www.inc.com/geoffrey-james/stop-working-more-than-40-hours-a-week.html. Accessed November 29, 2012.

7. Datamonitor, "Soaring Stress Levels Drive British Consumers to Splash Out on Premium Treats," October 14, 2004.

8. T.F. Heatherton and R.F. Baumeister, "Binge Eating as Escape from Self-awareness," *Psychology Bulletin* 110, no. 1 (July 1991): 86–108.

9. Health Canada website "About" page, http://www.hc-sc.gc.ca/ahc-asc/index-eng.php. Accessed July 19, 2013.

10. American Dietetic Association 2010 Annual Report: 6.

11. National Restaurant Association "About Us" website, http://www.restaurant.org/aboutus/whatwedo/. Accessed November 1, 2012.

12. Ibid.

13. "Ag Subsidies Pay for 21 Twinkies Per Taxpayer, but Only Half an Apple Apiece," Public Interest Research Group, https://www.uspirg.org/news/usp/ag-subsidies-pay-21-twinkies-taxpayer-only-half-apple-apiece. Accessed November 17, 2012.

14. Centers for Disease Control and Prevention, "The New (Ab) Normal," http://makinghealtheasier.org/newabnormal. Accessed March 6, 2013.

15. Jeremy Manier, Patricia Callahan and Delroy Alexander, "The Oreo, Obesity and Us," *Chicago Tribune*, August 21, 2005. Accessed online November 13, 2012.

16. Jeremy Manier, Patricia Callahan and Delroy Alexander, "Where There's Smoke, There Might Be Food Research Too," *Chicago Tribune*, January 29, 2006. Accessed online November 13, 2012.

17. Ibid.

18. H.I. Ziauddeen and P.C. Fletcher, "Obesity and the Brain: How Convincing Is the Addiction Model?" *Nature Reviews Neuroscience* 13, no. 4 (2012): 279–86.

2. WHY WE'RE FAT, PART 2—THE SCIENCE OF SIZE

1. Rudolph Leibel et al., "Energy Intake Required to Maintain Body Weight Is Not Affected by Wide Variation in Diet Composition," *American Journal of Clinical Nutrition* 55 (1992): 350–55.

2. A. Golay and E. Bobbioni, "The Role of Dietary Fat in Obesity," *International Journal of Obesity Related and Related Metabolic Disorders, Suppl 3*, June 1997: S2–11.

3. A. Buchholz and D. Schoeller, "Is a Calorie a Calorie?" *American Journal of Clinical Nutrition 79*, no. 5 (2004): 899S–906S.

4. D. Schoeller and A. Buchholz, "Energetics of Obesity and Weight Control: Does Diet Composition Matter?" *Journal of the American Dietetic Association 105* (5 Suppl 1), 2005: S24–28; K.R. Westerterp, "Physical Activity, Food Intake and Body Weight Regulation: Insights from Doubly-labeled Water Studies," *Nutrition Reviews 68*, no. 3 (2010): 148–54; T. Brown et al., "Systematic Review of Long-term Lifestyle Interventions to Prevent Weight Gain and Morbidity in Adults," *Obesity Reviews 10*, no. 6 (2009): 627–38; James Hill, "Understanding and Addressing the Epidemic of Obesity: An Energy Balance Perspective," *Endocrine Reviews 27*, no. 7 (2006): 750–61; L. Tappy, "Metabolic Consequences of Overfeeding in Humans," *Current Opinion and Medical Nutrition and Metabolic Care 7*, no. 6 (2004): 623–28; Annsi Manninen, "Is a Calorie Really a Calorie? Metabolic Advantage of Low-carbohydrate Diets," *Journal of the International Society of Sports Nutrition 1*, no. 2 (2004): 21–26; Manny Noakes et al., "Comparison of an Isocaloric Very Low Carbohydrate / High Saturated Fat and High Carbohydrate / Low Saturated Fat Diets on Body Composition and Cardiovascular Risk," *Nutrition and Metabolism 3*, no. 7 (2006): epub.

5. *This graphic was used with permission.* H.I. Ziauddeen and P.C. Fletcher, "Obesity and the Brain: How Convincing Is the Addiction Model?" *Nature Reviews Neuroscience 13*, no. 4 (2012): 279–86. The authors of this study also wish to pay credit to the Foresight program 2007, a multidisciplinary effort to plan the UK response to obesity. P. Vandenbroeck, J. Goossens and M. Clemens, *Tackling Obesities: Future Choices—Obesity System Atlas* (Government Office for Science, UK, 2007).

6. Caroline Fox et al., "Is a Low Leptin Concentration, a Low Resting Metabolic Rate, or Both the Expression of the 'Thrifty Genotype'?

Results from Mexican Pima Indians," *American Journal of Clinical Nutrition* 68 (1998): 1053; Claude Bouchard, ed., *Physical Activity and Obesity* (Champaign, IL: Human Kinetics, 2000), 13.

7. Nicole M. Avena et al., "Evidence for Sugar Addiction: Behavioral and Neurochemical Effects of Intermittent, Excessive Sugar Intake," *Neuroscience and Biobehavioural Reviews* 32, no. 1 (2008): 20–39; Nicole M. Avena, "Sucrose Sham Feeding on a Binge Schedule Releases Accumbens Dopamine Repeatedly and Eliminates the Acetylcholine Satiety Response," *Neuroscience* 139, no. 3 (2006): 813–20; P. Rada et al., "Daily Bingeing on Sugar Repeatedly Releases Dopamine in the Accumbens Shell," *Neuroscience* 134, no. 3 (2005): 737–44; Nora D. Volkow et al., "Overlapping Neuronal Circuits in Addiction and Obesity: Evidence of Systems Pathology," *Philosophical Transactions of the Royal Society of London B Biological Sciences* 363, no. 1507 (2008): 3191–3200; Gene Jack Wang et al., "Brain Dopamine and Obesity," *Lancet* 357, no. 9253 (2001): 354–57; Nora D. Volkow et al., "Reward, Dopamine and the Control of Food Intake: Implications for Obesity," *Trends in Cognitive Sciences* 15, no. 1 (2011): 37–46.

8. Kent C. Berridge et al., "The Tempted Brain Eats: Pleasure and Desire Circuits in Obesity and Eating Disorders," *Brain Research* 1350 (2010): 43–64; H. Berthoud et al., "Food Reward, Hyperphagia, and Obesity," *American Journal of Physiology* 300, no. 6 (2011): R1266–77.

9. P. Grigson, "Like Drugs for Chocolate: Separate Rewards Modulated by Common Mechanisms?" *Physiology and Behavior* 76, no. 3 (2002): 389–95; M. Yeomans and E. Coughlan, "Mood-Induced Eating: Interactive Effects of Restraint and Tendency to Overeat," *Appetite* 52, no. 2–3 (2009): 290–98; T. Van Strien et al., "Restraint, Tendency toward Overeating and Ice Cream Consumption," *International Journal of Eating Disorders* 28, no. 3 (2000): 333–38; A. Ruderman, "Dietary Restraint: A Theoretical and Empirical Review," *Psychological Bulletin* 99, no. 2 (1986): 247–62; A. Ruderman and H. Christensen, "Restraint Theory and

Its Applicability to Overweight Individuals," *Journal of Abnormal Psychology* 92 (1983): 210–15; J. Polivy et al., "The Effect of Deprivation on Food Cravings and Eating Behavior in Restrained and Unrestrained Eaters," *International Journal of Eating Disorders* 38, no. 4 (2005): 301–9; C. Herman and J. Polivy, "Anxiety, Restraint and Eating Behavior," *Journal of Abnormal Psychology* 84, no. 6 (1975): 66–72; K. Berridge, "Food Reward: Brain Substrates of Wanting and Liking," *Neuroscience and Biobehavioral Reviews* 20 (1996): 1–25.

10. Kent C. Berridge and Terry E. Robinson, "Parsing Reward," *Trends in Neuroscience* 26, no. 9 (2003): 507–13; S. Peciña and Kent C. Berridge, "Hedonic Hot Spot in Nucleus Accumbens Shell: Where Do Mu-opioids Cause Increased Hedonic Impact of Sweetness?" *Journal of Neuroscience* 25 (2005): 11777–86; Anne E. Kelley et al., "Neural Systems Recruited by Drug- and Food-related Cues: Studies of Gene Activation in Corticolimbic Regions," *Physiology and Behavior* 86, no. 1–2 (2005): 11–14; Anne E. Kelley et al., "Opioid Modulation of Taste Hedonics within the Ventral Striatum," *Physiology and Behavior* 76, no. 3 (2002): 365–77.

11. Ibid.; C. Erlanson-Albertsson, "How Palatable Food Disrupts Appetite Regulation," *Basic Clinical and Pharmacological Toxicology* 97, no. 2 (2005): 61–73; C. Erlanson-Albertsson, "Sugar Triggers Our Reward-System: Sweets Release Opiates Which Stimulates the Appetite for Sucrose—Insulin Can Depress It," *Lakartidningen* 192, no. 21 (2005): 1620–22, 1625, 1627.

12. K. Kamijo et al., "The Negative Association of Childhood Obesity to Cognitive Control of Action Monitoring," *Cerebral Cortex* (2012): epub ahead of print; K. McRae et al., "Bottom-up and Top-down Emotion Generation: Implications for Emotion Regulation," *Social Cognitive Affective Neuroscience* 7, no. 3 (2012): 253–62; J.M. Quinn, "Can't Control Yourself? Monitor Those Bad Habits," *Personality and Social Psychology Bulletin* 36, no. 4 (2010): 499–511; P. Dayan and B.W. Balleine, "Reward, Motivation, and Reinforcement Learning," *Neuron* 36, no. 2 (2002): 285–98.

13. Michael R. Lowe and M.L. Butryn, "Hedonic Hunger: A New Dimension of Appetite?" *Physiology and Behavior* 91, no. 4 (2007): 432–39; Michael R. Lowe and A.S. Levine, "Eating Motives and the Controversy over Dieting: Eating Less Than Needed versus Less Than Wanted," *Obesity Research* 13, no. 5 (2005): 797–806.

14. P.C. Konturek et al., "Neuro-hormonal Control of Food Intake: Basic Mechanisms and Clinical Implications," *Journal of Physiology and Pharmacology* 56, Suppl 6: 5–25; R.E. Nisbett, "Determinants of Food Intake in Obesity," *Science* 159, no. 820 (1968): 1254–55; G.N. Wade and I. Zucker, "Development of Hormonal Control over Food Intake and Body Weight in Female Rats," *Journal of Comparative Physiology and Psychology* 70, no. 2 (1970): 213–20; Hans Rudolph Berthoud and H. Munzberg, "The Lateral Hypothalamus as Integrator of Metabolic and Environmental Needs: From Electrical Self-stimulation to Opto-genetics," *Physiology and Behavior* 104, no. 1 (2011): 29–39; Hans-Rudolph Berthoud, "Interactions between the 'Cognitive' and 'Metabolic' Brain in the Control of Food Intake," *Physiology and Behavior* 91, no. 5 (2007): 486–98; A.P. Coll et al., "The Hormonal Control of Food Intake," *Cell* 129, no. 2 (2007): 251–62; M.O. Dietrich and T.L. Horvath, "Feeding Signals and Brain Circuitry," *European Journal of Neuroscience* 30, no. 9 (2009): 1688–96; A.P. Coll et al., "The Hormonal Control of Food Intake," *Cell* 129, no. 2 (2007): 251–62.

15. Lowe and Butryn, "Hedonic Hunger"; Lowe and Levine, "Eating Motives"; John E. Blundell and Graham Finlayson, "Is Susceptibility to Weight Gain Characterized by Homeostatic or Hedonic Risk Factors for Overconsumption?" *Physiology and Behavior* 82, no. 1 (2004): 21–25.

16. Lowe and Butryn, "Hedonic Hunger"; Lowe and Levine, "Eating Motives."

17. Kent C. Berridge, "Building a Neuroscience of Pleasure and Well-being," *Psychology of Well Being* 24, no. 1 (2011): 1–3; John E. Blundell et al., "Resistance and Susceptibility to Weight Gain: Individual Variability in Response to a High-fat Diet," *Physiology and*

Behavior 86, no. 5 (2005): 614–22; N. Pecoraro et al., "Chronic Stress Promotes Palatable Feeding, Which Reduces Signs of Stress: Feed Forward and Feedback Effects of Chronic Stress," *Endocrinology* 145 (2003): 3745–62.

18. K. Blum et al., "Sex, Drugs, and Rock 'n' Roll: Hypothesizing Common Mesolimbic Activation as a Function of Reward Gene Polymorphisms," *Journal of Psychoactive Drugs* 44, no. 1 (2012): 38–55; Berridge, "Building a Neuroscience of Pleasure and Well-being"; W.A.Wilson, "The Role of Learning, Perception and Reward in Monkeys' Choice of Food," *American Journal of Psychology* 72 (1959): 560–65; Berridge and Robinson, "Parsing Reward."

19. Ibid.; M.G.D. Le Moal and B. Cardo, "Behavioral Effects of Local Injection of 6-Hydroxydopamine in the Medial Ventral Tegmentum in the Rat: Possible Role of the Mesolimbic Dopamingergic System," *Brain Research* 88, no. 1 (1975): 190–94; K.W. Blum et al., "Sex, Drugs, and Rock 'n' Roll."

20. J.A. Nasser et al., "Psychoactive Effects of Tasting Chocolate and Desire for More Chocolate," *Physiology and Behavior* 104, no. 1 (2011): 117–21.

21. Peciña and Berridge, "Hedonic Hot Spot in Nucleus Accumbens Shell."

22. Nasser et al., "Psychoactive Effects of Tasting Chocolate and Desire for More Chocolate."

23. J.A. Cocores, "The Salted Food Addiction Hypothesis May Explain Overeating and the Obesity Epidemic," *Medical Hypothesis* 73, no. 6 (2009): 892–99.

24. Ibid.

25. Berridge and Robinson, "Parsing Reward."

26. Wilson, "The Role of Learning, Perception, and Reward in Monkeys' Choice of Food"; Erlanson-Albertsson, "Sugar Triggers Our Reward-system"; Erlanson-Albertsson, "How Palatable Food Disrupts Appetite Regulation"; Nicole M. Avena et al., "Evidence for Sugar Addiction"; Nicole M. Avena, "Sucrose Sham Feeding on

a Binge Schedule Releases Accumbens Dopamine Repeatedly and Eliminates the Acetylcholine Satiety Response"; Hans Rudolph Berthoud, "Food Reward, Hyperphagia and Obesity," *American Journal of Physiology Regulatory Integrative and Comparative Physiology* 300, no. 6 (2011): R1266–77.

27. Caroline A. Davis et al., "Dopamine for 'Wanting' and Opioids for 'Liking': A Comparison of Obese Adults with and without Binge Eating," *Obesity*, 17, no. 6 (2009): 1220–5; Kent C. Berridge and Terry E. Robinson, "What Is the Role of Dopamine in Reward: Hedonic Impact, Reward Learning, or Incentive Salience?" *Brain Research Reviews* 28, no. 3 (1998): 309–69.

28. K. D'Ardenne et al., "Role of Prefrontal Cortex and the Midbrain Dopamine System in Working Memory Updating," *Procedures of the National Academy of Science U.S.A.*, October 2012 epub ahead of print; T. Sawaguchi et al., "Dopamine Enhances the Neuronal Activity of Spatial Short-term Memory Task in the Primate Prefrontal Cortex," *Neuroscience Research* 5, no. 5 (1988): 465–73.

29. Kelley et al., "Opioid Modulation of Taste Hedonics within the Ventral Striatum"; Kelley et al., "Neural Systems Recruited by Drug- and Food-related Cues."

30. Davis et al., "Dopamine for 'Wanting' and Opioids for 'Liking.' "

31. P.K. Olszewski et al., "Opioids as Facilitators of Feeding: Can Any Food Be Rewarding?" *Physiology and Behavior* 104, no. 1 (2011): 105–110.

32. Kelley et al., "Opioid Modulation"; Kelley et al., "Neural Systems."

33. W. Michener and W.P. Rozin, "Pharmacological versus Sensory Factors in the Satiation of Chocolate Craving," *Physiology and Behavior* 56 (1994): 419–22; J.L. Osman and J. Sobal, "Chocolate Cravings in American and Spanish Individuals: Biological and Cultural Influences," *Appetite* 47 (2006): 290–301.

34. P. Rada et al., "Opioids in the Hypothalamus Control Dopamine and Acetylcholine Levels in the Nucleus Accumbens," *Brain Research* 1312 (2010): 1–9; Anne E. Kelley et al., "A Pharmacological Analysis of the Substrates Underlying Conditioned Feeding

Induced by Repeated Opioid Stimulation of the Nucleus Accumbens," *Neuropsychopharmacology* 23, no. 4 (2000): 455–67.

35. Nora D. Volkow et al., "Reward, Dopamine and the Control of Food Intake: Implications for Obesity," *Trends in Cognitive Science* 15, no. 1 (2011): 37–46; Rada et al., "Daily Bingeing on Sugar Repeatedly Releases Dopamine in the Accumbens Shell"; P.J. Nathan and E.T. Bullmore, "From Taste Hedonics to Motivational Drive: Central μ-Opioid Receptors and Binge-eating Behaviour," *International Journal of Neuropsychopharmacology* 12, no. 7 (2009): 995–1008; G. DiChiara, "Dopamine in Disturbances of Food and Drug Motivated Behavior: A Case of Homology?" *Physiology and Behavior* 86, no. 1–2 (2005): 9–10.

36. Ibid.

37. Gene-Jack Wang et al., "Brain Dopamine and Obesity," *Lancet* 357, no. 9253 (2001): 354–57; Volkow et al., "Overlapping Neuronal Circuits in Addiction and Obesity: Evidence of Systems Pathology."

38. Wang et al., "Brain Dopamine."

39. K.S. Burger and E. Stice, "Frequent Ice Cream Consumption Is Associated with Reduced Striatal Response to Receipt of an Ice Cream–Based Milkshake," *American Journal of Clinical Nutrition* 95, no. 4 (2012): 810–17.

40. Molly Crocket et al., "Restricting Temptations: Neural Mechanisms of Precommitment," *Neuron* 79, no. 2 (2013): 391–401.

41. Barbara J. Rolls, "Sensory-specific Satiety," *Nutrition Review* 44, no. 3 (1986): 93–101.

42. Ibid.

43. Barbara J. Rolls et al., "Pleasantness Changes and Food Intake in a Varied Four-course Meal," *Appetite* 5, no. 4 (1984): 337–48; Barbara J. Rolls et al., "Variety in the Diet Enhances Intake in a Meal and Contributes to the Development of Obesity in the Rat," *Physiology and Behavior* 31, no. 1 (1983): 21–27; Rolls, "Sensory-specific Satiety"; S.L. Tey et al., "Long-term Consumption of High Energy-dense Snack Foods on Sensory-specific Satiety and Intake," *American Journal of Clinical Nutrition* 95, no. 5 (2012): 1038–47.

44. I.C. Macedo et al., "Cafeteria Diet–Induced Obesity Plus Chronic Stress Alter Serum Leptin Levels," *Peptides* 38, no. 1 (2012): 189–96.

45. Mary M. Boggiano et al., "The Pavlovian Power of Palatable Food: Lessons for Weight-loss Adherence from a New Rodent Model of Cue-induced Overeating," *International Journal of Obesity* 33, no. 6 (2009): 693–701.

46. Volkow et al., "Overlapping Neuronal Circuits in Addiction and Obesity"; Boggiano et al., "The Pavlovian Power of Palatable Food."

47. H. Ziauddeen et al., "Food Images Engage Subliminal Motivation to Seek Food," *International Journal of Obesity* 36, no. 9 (2012): 1245–47; Natalie S. Lawrence et al., "Nucleus Accumbens Response to Food Cues Predicts Subsequent Snack Consumption in Women and Increased Body Mass Index in Those with Reduced Self-control," *Neuroimage* 63 (2012): 415–22.

48. S. Söderqvist et al., "Dopamine, Working Memory and Training Induced Plasticity: Implications for Developmental Research," *Developmental Psychology* 48, no. 3 (2012): 836–43; V.S. Störmer, "Dopaminergic and Cholinergic Modulations of Visual-spatial Attention and Working Memory: Insights from Molecular Genetic Research and Implications for Adult Cognitive Development," *Developmental Psychology* 48, no. 3 (2012): 875–89.

49. G.D. Petrovich, "Learning and the Motivation to Eat: Forebrain Circuitry," *Physiology and Behavior* 104, no. 4 (2011): 582–89; J.D. Beaver, "Individual Differences in Reward Drive Predict Neural Responses to Images of Food," *Journal of Neuroscience* 26, no. 19 (2006): 5160–66.

50. D. Gaillard et al., "Molecular Mechanisms of Fat Preference and Overeating," *Annual New York Academy of Science* 1141 (2008): 163–75.

51. Boggiano et al., "The Pavlovian Power of Palatable Food."

52. Ibid.

53. Lawrence et al., "Nucleus Accumbens Response to Food Cues"; J.D. Beaver et al., "Individual Differences in Reward Drive Predict Neural Responses to Images of Food," *Journal of Neuroscience* 26, no. 19 (2006): 5160–66.

54. Kent C. Berridge et al., "The Tempted Brain Eats: Pleasure and Desire Circuits in Obesity and Eating Disorders," *Brain Research* 1350 (2010): 43–64.

55. R. Cornell and Harvey Weingarten, "Stimulus-induced Eating When Satiated," *Physiology and Behavior* 45 (1989): 695–704.

56. Email from Emma Boyland, research associate in experimental psychology, University of Liverpool, to Margaret Yúfera-Leitch, 2012.

57. R.M. Piech et al., "All I Saw Was the Cake: Hunger Effects on Attentional Capture by Visual Food Cues," *Appetite* 54, no. 3 (2010): 579–82.

58. Lawrence et al., "Nucleus Accumbens Response to Food Cues."

59. Leonard H. Epstein et al., "Food Reinforcement and Obesity. Psychological Moderators," *Appetite* 58, no. 1 (2012): 157–62; Leonard H. Epstein, "Food Reinforcement, Delay Discounting and Obesity," *Physiology and Behavior* 100, no. 5 (2010): 438–45; Leonard H. Epstein, "Habituation as a Determinant of Human Food Intake," *Psychology Reviews* 116, no. 2 (2009): 384–407.

60. Boggiano et al., "The Pavlovian Power of Palatable Food"; R.A. Wise, "Role of Brain Dopamine in Food Reward and Reinforcement," *Philosophical Transactions of the Royal Society of London B Biological Sciences* 361, no. 1149 (2006): 1149–58.

61. Terry E. Robinson and Kent C. Berridge, "Incentive-sensitization and Addiction," *Addiction* 96, no. 1 (2001): 103–14; Terry E. Robinson and Kent C. Berridge, "Addiction," *Annual Reviews of Psychology* 54 (2003): 25–53.

62. Ibid.

63. Kent C. Berridge, "Wanting and Liking: Observations from the Neuroscience and Psychology Laboratory," *Inquiry* 52, no. 4 (2009): 378; Berridge and Robinson, "Parsing Reward."

64. W.J. Rejeski et al., "State Craving, Food Availability, and Reactivity to Preferred Snack Foods," *Appetite* 54, no. 1 (2010): 77–83.

65. Ibid.

66. Bart G. Hoebel, "Inhibition and Disinhibition of Self-stimulation and Feeding: Hypothalamic Control and Postingestional Factors," *Computational Physiology and Psychology* 66 (1968): 89–100.

67. Lawrence et al., "Nucleus Accumbens Response to Food Cues"; K.D. Carr, "Chronic Food Restriction: Enhancing Effects on Drug Reward and Striatal Cell Signaling," *Physiology and Behavior* 91, no. 5 (2012): 459–72; K.D. Carr, "Food Scarcity, Neuroadaptations, and the Pathogenic Potential of Dieting in an Unnatural Ecology: Binge Eating and Drug Abuse," *Physiology and Behavior* 104, no. 1 (2011): 162–67.

68. L.H. Sweet et al., "Brain Response to Food Stimulation in Obese, Normal Weight, and Successful Weight Loss Maintainers," *Obesity* 20, no. 11 (2012): 2220–25.

69. M.A. Cornier et al., "The Effects of Exercise on the Neuronal Response to Food Cues," *Physiology and Behavior* 105, no. 4 (2012): 1028–34.

70. Ibid.

71. "Risks and Benefits of Alcohol Consumption," *Alcohol Research and Health* 24, no. 1 (2000): 5–11.

72. Mahmoud El-Sayed et al., "Interaction between Alcohol and Exercise: Physiological and Haematological Implications," *Sports Medicine* 35, no. 3 (2005): 257–69.

73. Ibid.

74. Samara Joy Nielsen et al., "Calories Consumed from Alcohol Beverages by U.S. Adults, 2007–2010," National Center for Health Statistics Data Brief No. 110, Centers for Disease Control and Prevention, November 2012.

75. Emannuelle Kesse et al., "Do Eating Habits Differ According to Alcohol Consumption?: Results of a Study of the French Cohort of the European Prospective Investigation into Cancer and Nutrition," *American Journal of Clinical Nutrition* 74, no. 3 (September 2001): 322–27.

76. Marion Hetherington et al., "Stimulation of Appetite by Alcohol," *Physiology and Behavior* 74, no. 3 (2001): 283–89; Eleanor Bryant et al., "Disinhibition: Its Effects on Appetite and Weight Regulation," *Obesity Reviews* 9, no. 5 (September 2008): 409–19; M.R. Yeomans et al., "Alcohol and the Appetizer Effect," *Behavioural Pharmacology* 10,

no. 2 (1999): 151–61; M.R. Yeomans, "Effects of Alcohol on Food and Energy Intake in Human Subjects: Evidence for Passive and Active Over-consumption of Energy," *British Journal of Nutrition* 92, suppl.1 (August 2004): S31–34.

3. WHY YOU SHOULD BE EXCITED TO CHANGE

1. Albert Bandura, "Self-efficacy: Toward a Unifying Theory of Behavioral Change," *Psychological Review* 84 (March 1977): 191–215.
2. Vasilios Kosteas, "The Effect of Exercise on Earnings: Evidence from the NLSY," *Journal of Labor Research* 33 (June 2012): 225–50.
3. J.B. Dixon et al., International Diabetes Federation Taskforce on Epidemiology and Prevention. "Bariatric Surgery: An IDF Statement for Obese Type 2 Diabetes," *Diabetes Medicine* 28, no. 6 (June 2011): 628–42.
4. Brenda Major et al., "The Psychological Weight of Weight Stigma," *Social Psychological and Personality Science* 3 (November 2012): 651–58.
5. Angelina Sutin and Antonio Terracciano, "Perceived Weight Discrimination and Obesity," *PLoS ONE* 8(7) (July 2013): e70048.
6. Claude Bouchard, ed., *Physical Activity and Obesity* (Champaign, IL: Human Kinetics, 2000), 3; George Bray, "Overweight, Mortality and Morbidity," *Physical Activity and Obesity*: 31.
7. Martin Hagger and Nikos Chatzisarantis, *The Social Psychology of Exercise and Sport* (New York: Open University Press, 2005), 8–9.
8. Edward Gregg et al., "Secular Trends in Cardiovascular Disease Risk Factors According to Body Mass Index in U.S. Adults," *Journal of the American Medical Association* 293, no. 15 (April 20, 2005): 1868–74.
9. Hagger and Chatzisarantis, *Social Psychology of Exercise and Sport*, 8–9.
10. Timothy Church et al., "Exercise Capacity and Body Composition as Predictors of Mortality among Men with Diabetes," *Diabetes Care* 27, no. 1 (January 2004): 83–88; Peter Katzmarzyk et al., "Metabolic Syndrome, Obesity and Mortality," *Diabetes Care* 28, no. 2

(February 2005): 391–97; Chong Do Lee et al., "Cardiorespiratory Fitness, Body Composition, and All-cause Cardiovascular Disease Mortality in Men," *American Journal of Clinical Nutrition* 69 (March 1999): 373–80; Gail Marchessault, "Obesity in Manitoba Adults," University of Manitoba Faculty of Medicine, October 2011.

11. K.M. Flegal et al., "Association of All-cause Mortality with Overweight and Obesity Using Standard Body Mass Index Categories: A Systematic Review and Meta-analysis," *Journal of the American Medical Association* 309, no. 1 (January 2, 2013): 71–82.

12. E.E. Calle et al., "Body-mass Index and Mortality in a Prospective Cohort of U.S. Adults," *New England Journal of Medicine* 341, no. 15 (October 7, 1999): 1097–1105.

13. C.H. Hennekens and F. Andreotti, "Leading Avoidable Cause of Premature Deaths Worldwide: Case for Obesity," *American Journal of Medicine* 126, no. 2 (February 2013): epub.

14. Curt Lox et al., *The Psychology of Exercise: Integrating Theory and Practice* (Scottsdale, AZ: Holcomb Hathaway, 2006), 27.

15. Pranesh Chowdhery et al., "Surveillance of Certain Health Behaviors and Conditions Among States and Selected Local Areas—Behavioral Risk Factor Surveillance System, United States, 2007," http://www.cdc.gov/mmwr/preview/mmwrhtml/ss5901a1.htm. Accessed November 17, 2012.

16. Ian Janssen et al., "Fitness Alters the Associations of BMI and Waist Circumference with Total and Abdominal Fat," *Obesity* 12, no. 3 (2012): 525–37; L.B. Andersen et al., "Fitness, Fatness and Clustering of Cardiovascular Risk Factors in Children from Denmark, Estonia and Portugal: The European Youth Heart Study," *International Journal of Pediatric Obesity* 3 (2008): 58–66; Chiung-ju Liu and Nancy Latham, "Progressive Resistance Strength Training for Improving Physical Function in Older Adults," *Cochrane Library*, July 8, 2009; Pierpaulo De Feo et al., "Physical Inactivity Is the Main Cause of Metabolic Syndrome," in *Role of Physical Exercise in Preventing Disease and Improving the Quality of Life*, ed. Vilberto Stocchi et al. (Milan: Springer-Verlag,

2007), 30; Kay-Tee Khaw et al., "Combined Impact of Health Behaviors and Mortality in Men and Women: The EPIC-Norfolk Prospect Population Study," *PLoS Medicine* 5, no. 1 (January 2008): epub; L. Ferrucci et al., "Smoking, Physical Activity and Active Life Expectancy," *American Journal of Epidemiology* 149, no. 7 (1999): 645–53; Juha Pekkanen et al., "Reduction of Premature Mortality by High Physical Activity: A 20-Year Follow-up of Middle-aged Finnish Men," *Lancet,* June 27, 1987: 1473–77; Dellara Terry et al., "Disentangling the Roles of Disability and Morbidity in Survival to Exceptional Old Age," *Archives of Internal Medicine* 168, no. 3 (February 11, 2008): 277–83; David Hood et al., "Exercise-induced Mitochondrial Biogenesis in Skeletal Muscle," in *Role of Physical Exercise,* 52; Michele Guescini et al., "Molecular Modifications Induced by Physical Exercise: A Significant Role in Disease Prevention," in *Role of Physical Exercise,* 94.

17. K. Esposito et al., "Obesity and Sexual Dysfunction, Male and Female," *International Journal of Impotence Research* 20, no. 4 (July–August 2008): 358–65.

18. Terry et al., "Disentangling the Roles of Disability and Morbidity."

19. Ruth Ann Atchley et al., "Creativity in the Wild: Improving Creative Reasoning through Immersion in Natural Settings," *PLoS ONE* 7, no. 12 (December 2012): epub.

4. WHY YOU *MUST* EXERCISE

1. Michelle Voss et al., "Exercise, Brain, and Cognition across the Life Span," *Journal of Applied Physiology* 111, no. 5 (2011): 1505–13.

2. Albertine Schuit et al., "Physical Activity and Cognitive Decline: The Role of the Apoliproprotein e4 Allele," *Medicine and Science in Sports and Exercise* 33, no. 5 (May 2001): 772–77.

3. J.Z. Wiley et al., "Lower Prevalence of Silent Brain Infarcts in the Physically Active: The Northern Manhattan Study," *Neurology* 76, no. 24 (June 2011): 2112–18.

4. A. Tsatsoulis and S. Fountoulakis, "The Protective Role of Exercise on Stress System Dysregulation and Comorbidities," *Annals of the New York Academy of Sciences* 1083 (November 2006): 196–213.

5. Ibid.

6. Ibid.

7. "Exercise for Stress and Anxiety," http://www.adaa.org/living-with-anxiety/managing-anxiety/exercise-stress-and-anxiety. Accessed November 23, 2012.

8. R. Stark et al., "Acute Effects of a Single Bout of Moderate Exercise on Psychological Well-being in Patients with Affective Disorder during Hospital Treatment," *Neuropsychiatry*, October 2012: epub ahead of print; A.M. Lane and D.J. Lovejoy, "The Effects of Exercise on Mood Changes: The Moderating Effect of Depressed Mood," *Journal of Sports Medicine and Physical Fitness* 41, no. 4 (December 2001): 539–45; A.M. Lane et al., "Mood Changes Following Exercise," *Perception and Motor Skills* 94, no. 3, pt. 1 (June 2002): 732–34; T.W. Scheewe et al., "Exercise Therapy Improves Mental and Physical Health in Schizophrenia: A Randomized Control Trial," *Acta Psychiatra Scandanavia*, epub ahead of print; Martin Kopp et al., "Acute Effects of Brisk Walking on Affect and Psychological Well-being in Individuals with Type 2 Diabetes," *Diabetes Research and Clinical Practice* 95, no. 1 (January 2012): 25–29; Madhukar Trivedi et al., "Exercise as an Augmentation Strategy for Treatment of Major Depression," *Journal of Psychiatric Practice* 12, no. 4 (2006): 205–13; K. Martiny et al., "A 9-Week Randomized Trial Comparing a Chronotherapeutic Intervention (Wake and Light Therapy) to Exercise in Major Depressive Disorder Patients Treated with Duloxetine," *Journal of Clinical Psychiatry* 73, no. 9 (September 2012): 1234–42; J. Mata et al., "Acute Exercise Attenuates Negative Affect Following Repeated Sad Mood Inductions in Persons Who Have Recovered from Depression," *Journal of Abnormal Psychology*, 2012: epub ahead of print; J.B. Bartholomew et al., "Effects of Acute Exercise on Mood and Well-being in Patients with Major

Depressive Disorder," *Medicine and Science in Sports and Exercise* 37, no. 12 (2005): 2032–37.

9. Jennifer L. Steiner et al., "Exercise Training Increases Mitochondrial Biogenesis in the Brain," *Journal of Applied Physiology* 111, no. 4 (October 2011): 1066–71.

10. Brian Wansink, *Mindless Eating: Why We Eat More Than We Think* (New York: Bantam, 2010), 1.

11. R.J. Joseph et al., "The Neurocognitive Connection between Physical Activity and Eating Behavior," *Obesity Reviews* 12, no. 19 (October 2011): 800–812.

12. Maciej Buchowski et al., "Aerobic Exercise Training Reduces Cannabis Craving and Use in Non-treatment Seeking Cannabis-Dependent Adults," *PLoS ONE* 6, no. 3 (March 2011): e17465.

13. Mark Smith and Wendy Lynch, "Exercise as a Potential Treatment for Drug Abuse: Evidence from Preclinical Studies," *Frontiers in Psychiatry* 82, no. 2 (January 2012): 1–10.

14. K.A. Krawczewski, "Voluntary Exercise Improves High-fat Diet-induced Leptin Resistance Independent of Adiposity," *Endocrinology* 152, no. 7 (July 2011): 2655–64.

15. C. Martins, "Effects of Exercise and Restrained Eating Behaviour on Appetite Control," *Procedures of the Nutrition Society* 67, no. 1 (February 2008): 28–41; C. Martins et al., "Short-term Appetite Control in Response to a 6-Week Exercise Program in Sedentary Volunteers," *British Journal of Nutrition* 98, no. 4 (2007): 834–42; B. Hanlon et al., "Neural Response to Pictures of Food after Exercise in Normal and Obese Women," *Medical Sports Exercise* 44, no. 10 (2012): 1864–70; N. Evero et al., "Aerobic Exercise Reduces Neuronal Responses in Food Reward Brain Regions," *Journal of Applied Physiology* 112, no. 9 (2012): 1612–19.

16. K.J. Guelfi et al., "Beneficial Effects of 12 Weeks of Aerobic Compared with Resistance Exercise Training on Perceived Appetite in Previously Sedentary Overweight and Obese Men," *Metabolism*, September 2012: epub ahead of print.

17. A.Y. Sim et al., "High-Intensity Intermittent Exercise Attenuates

Ad-libitum Energy Intake," *International Journal of Obesity*, July 2013: epub ahead of print; D. Ennette Larson-Meyer et al., "Influence of Running and Walking on Hormonal Regulators of Appetite in Women," *Journal of Obesity*, 2012: 1–15.

18. K. Granados et al., "Appetite Regulation in Response to Sitting and Energy Imbalance," *Applied Physiology, Nutrition, and Metabolism* 37, no. 2 (2012): 323–33.

19. S. Hattori et al., "Striatal Dopamine Turnover during Treadmill Running in the Rat: Relation to the Speed of Running," *Brain Research Bulletin* 35, no. 1 (1994): 41–49.

20. S.J. O'Dell et al., "Running Wheel Exercise Ameliorates Methamphetamine-induced Damage to Dopamine and Serotonin Terminals," *Synapse* 66, no. 1 (2012): 71–80.

21. Michelle Tucker and Marla Reicks, "Exercise as a Gateway Behavior for Healthful Eating among Older Adults: An Exploratory Study," *Journal of Nutrition Education and Behavior* 34, S1 (March–April 2002): S14–19; Edwin Boudreaux, "Congruence of Readiness to Change, Self-efficacy, and Decisional Balance for Physical Activity and Dietary Fat Reduction," *American Journal of Health Promotion* 17, no. 5 (May–June 2003): 329–36.

22. "Brain Scans Show Specific Neuronal Response to Junk Food When Sleep-restricted," American Academy of Sleep Medicine News Archive, June 10, 2012.

23. C. Benedict, "Acute Sleep Deprivation Enhances the Brain's Response to Hedonic Food Stimuli: An fMRI Study," *Journal of Clinical Endocrinology and Metabolism* 97, no. 3 (2012): E443; Marie-Pierre St.-Onge, "Sleep Restriction Leads to Increased Activation of Brain Regions Sensitive to Food Stimuli," *American Society for Nutrition* 95, no. 4 (2012): 818–24.

24. Julie Shlisky et al., "Partial Sleep Deprivation and Energy Balance in Adults: An Emerging Issue for Consideration by Dietetics Practitioners," *Journal of the Academy of Nutrition and Dietetics* 112, no. 11 (2012): 1785–97; Kathryn Reid et al., "Aerobic Exercise Improves Self-reported Sleep and Quality of Life in Older Adults

with Insomnia," *Sleep Medicine* 11, no. 9 (2012): 934–40; Nalin Singh et al., "A Randomized Controlled Trial of the Effect of Exercise on Sleep," *Sleep* 20, no. 2 (1997): 95–101; Shelley Tworoger et al., "Effects of a Yearlong Moderate-intensity Exercise and a Stretching Intervention on Sleep Quality in Postmenopausal Women," *Sleep* 26, no. 7 (2003): 830–36; Abby King et al., "Moderate-intensity Exercise and Self-rated Quality of Sleep in Older Adults: A Randomized Controlled Trial," *Journal of the American Medical Association* 277, no. 1 (January 1997): 32–37; David Buchner, "Physical Activity and Quality of Life in Older Adults," *Journal of the American Medical Association* 277, no. 1 (January 1997): 64–66; I.Vuori, "Epidemiology of Exercise Effects on Sleep," *Acta Physiologica Scandinavica*, suppl., 574 (1988): 3–7.

25. O. Werle et al., "Just Thinking about Exercise Makes Me Serve More Food: Physical Activity and Caloric Compensation," *Appetite* 56, no. 2 (April 2011): 332–35.

5. GET SMART: METABOLISM MYTH BUSTING

1. Jenni, "By George," http://aiyh.blogspot.ca/2005/06/by-george.html. Accessed November 20, 2012.

2. Laura Ries, "Jorge Cruise," April 2005, http://ries.typepad.com/ries_blog/2005/04/jorge_cruise.html. Accessed November 20, 2012.

3. National Weight Control Registry, http://www.nwcr.ws/Research/default.htm. Accessed November 10, 2012.

4. Ibid.; J.G. Thomas and R.R. Wing, "Maintenance of Long-Term Weight Loss," *Medical Health Reviews* 92, no. 2 (February 2009): 56–57.

5. Thomas Wadden et al., "Four-year Weight Losses in the Look AHEAD Study: Factors Associated with Long-term Success," *Obesity* 19, no. 10 (2011): 1987–98.

6. Claude Bouchard et al., *Genetics of Fitness and Physical Performance* (Champaign, IL: Human Kinetics, 1997), 189–90.

7. Darcy Johannsen et al., "Metabolic Slowing with Massive Weight Loss despite Preservation of Fat-free Mass," *Journal of Clinical Endocrinology and Metabolism* 97, no. 7 (2012): 2489–96.

8. David Perlmutter, "The Surprising Way Grains are Destroying Your Brain," August 28, 2013 at http://www.mindbodygreen.com/0-10753/the-surprising-ways-grains-are-destroying-your-brain.html. Accessed September 14, 2013.

9. World Health Organization, "Facts and Figures about Tobacco," February 2006: http://www.who.int/tobacco/fctc/tobacco%20 factsheet%20for%20COP4.pdf. Accessed September 14, 2013.

10. Michael Pollan, *In Defense of Food: An Eater's Manifesto* (New York: Penguin, 2008).

11. David Katz, "Separation of Church and Plate," *Huffington Post*, March 20, 2012: http://www.huffingtonpost.com/david-katz-md/ diets_b_1358147.html. Accessed September 14, 2013.

12. David Katz, "Can We Say What Diet Is 'Best'?" *Huffington Post*, September 7, 2011: http://www.huffingtonpost.com/david-katz-md/best-diets_b_950672.html. Accessed September 14, 2013.

13. G. Haff et al., "Carbohydrate Supplementation and Resistance Training," *Journal of Strength and Conditioning Research* 17(1) (2003): 187–86; P. Macdermid and S. Stannard, "A Whey-supplemented, High-protein Diet versus a High-carbohydrate Diet: Effects on Endurance Cycling Performance," *International Journal of Sport Nutrition and Exercise Metabolism* 16(1) (2006): 65–77; D. Christensen et al., "Food and Macronutrient Intake of Male Adolescent Kalenjin Runners in Kenya," *British Journal of Nutrition* 88(6) (2002): 711–717; L. Burke et al., "Carbohydrates for Training and Competition," *Journal of Sports Science,* 29 Supple (2011): epub ahead of print; R. Keith et al., "Alterations in Dietary Carbohydrate, Protein, and Fat Intake and Mood State in Trained Female Cyclists," *Medicine and Science in Sports and Exercise* 23(2) (1991): 2121–26; T. Vandenbogaerde and W. Hopkins, "Effects of Acute Carbohydrate Supplementation on Endurance Performance: A Meta-analysis," *Sports Medicine* 41(9) (2011): epub ahead of print;

J. Helge, "Adaptation to a Fat-rich Diet: Effects on Endurance Performance in Humans," *Sports Medicine* 30(5) (2000): 347–57; A. Lima-Silva et al., "Effects of a Low- or a High-carbohydrate Diet on Performance, Energy System Contribution, and Metabolic Responses during Supramaximal Exercise," *Applied Physiology, Nutrition and Metabolism* 38(9) (2013): epub ahead of print; N. Cermak and L. van Loon, "The Use of Carbohydrates during Exercise as an Ergogenic Aid," *Sports Medicine,* July 2013: epub ahead of print; J. Langfort et al., "The Effect of a Low-carbohydrate Diet on Performance, Hormonal and Metabolic Responses to a 30-s Bout of Supramaximal Exercise," *European Journal of Applied Physiology and Occupational Physiology* 76(2) (1997): 128–33.

6. GET REAL: CHANGING HOW YOU VIEW FOOD

1. Julia Ello-Martin et al., "The Influence of Food Portion Size and Energy Density on Energy Intake: Implications for Weight Management," *American Journal of Clinical Nutrition* 82, suppl. (2005): 236S–41S; Julia Ello-Martin et al., "Dietary Energy Density in the Treatment of Obesity: A Year-long Trial Comparing Two Weight-loss Diets," *American Journal of Clinical Nutrition* 85 (2007): 1465–77; Barbara Rolls et al., "Salad and Satiety: Energy Density and Portion Size of a First-course Salad Affect Energy Intake at Lunch," *Journal of the American Dietetic Association* 104 (2004): 1570; Jenny Ledikwe et al., "Dietary Energy Density Is Associated with Energy Intake and Weight Status in US Adults," *American Journal of Clinical Nutrition* 83 (2006): 1362; Jenny Ledikwe et al., "Reductions in Dietary Energy Density Are Associated with Weight Loss in Overweight and Obese Participants in the PREMIER Trial," *American Journal of Clinical Nutrition* 85 (2007): 1212; Jenny Ledikwe et al., "Low-energy-density Diets Are Associated with High Diet Quality in Adults in the United States," *Journal of the American Dietetic Association* 106 (2006): 1172.

2. Julie Flood et al., "The Effect of Increased Beverage Portion Size on Energy Intake at a Meal," *Journal of the American Dietetic Association* 106 (2006): 1984–90.

3. "Disinterested in Snacking: Quebecers Indulge in Dessert 30 Per Cent More than the Rest of Canadians," November 6, 2012. https://www.npdgroup.ca/wps/portal/npd/ca/news/canadas-slimmest-province-doesnt-shy-away-from-dessert/. Accessed November 20, 2012.

4. France Bellisle, "Impact of the Daily Meal Pattern on Energy Balance," *Scandinavian Journal of Nutrition* 48, no. 3 (2004): 114–18.

5. Bill Phillips and Michael D'Orso, *Body for Life: 12 Weeks to Mental and Physical Strength* (New York: HarperCollins, 1999), 44.

6. Bellisle, "Impact of the Daily Meal Pattern on Energy Balance."

7. Abdul Dulloo and Jean Jacquet, "Adaptive Reduction in Basal Metabolic Rate in Response to Food Deprivation in Humans: A Role for Feedback Signals from Fat Stores," *American Journal of Clinical Nutrition* 68 (1998): 599–606.

8. Abdul Dulloo et al., "Poststarvation Hyperphagia and Body Fat Overshooting in Humans: A Role for Feedback Signals from Lean and Fat Tissues," *American Journal of Clinical Nutrition* 65 (1997): 717–23.

9. Carla Miller et al., "Comparative Effectiveness of a Mindful Eating Intervention to a Diabetes Self-management Intervention among Adults with Type 2 Diabetes: A Pilot Study," *Journal of the Academy of Nutrition and Dietetics* 112, no. 11 (November 2012): 1835–42; R.C. Baker et al., "Weight Control during the Holidays: Highly Consistent Self-monitoring as a Potentially Useful Coping Mechanism," *Health Psychology* 17, no. 4 (July 1998): 367–70.

10. M.R. Yeomans, "Palatability and the Micro-structure of Feeding in Humans: The Appetizer Effect," *Appetite* 27, no. 2 (October 1996): 119–33; C. De Graaf et al., "Palatability Affects Satiation but Not Satiety," *Physiology and Behavior* 66, no. 4 (June 1999): 681–88; M.O. Monneuse, "Responses to an Intense Sweetener in Humans: Immediate Preference and Delayed Effects on Intake,"

Physiology and Behavior 49, no. 2 (February 1991): 325–30; E.M. Bobroff et al., "Effects in Changes of Palatability of Food Intake and the Cumulative Food Intake Curve in Man," *Appetite* 7, no. 1 (March 1986): 85–96; M.R. Yeomans et al., "Independent Effects of Palatability and Within-meal Pauses on Intake and Appetite Ratings in Human Volunteers," *Appetite* 29, no. 1 (August 1997): 61–76; L.B. Sørensen et al., "Effect of Sensory Perceptions of Foods on Appetite and Food Intake: A Review of Studies on Humans," *International Journal of Obesity and Related Metabolic Disorders* 27, no. 10 (October 2003): 1152–66; C. Hill et al., "The Relative Reinforcing Value of Food Predicts Weight Gain in a Longitudinal Study of 7–10-year-old Children," *American Journal of Clinical Nutrition* 90, no. 2 (August 2009): 276–81; E. Stice et al., "Reward Circuitry Responsivity to Food Predicts Future Increases in Body Mass: Moderating Effects of DRD2 and DRD4," *Neuroimage* 50, no. 4 (May 2010): 1618–25; S. Yokum et al., "Attentional Bias to Food Images Associated with Elevated Weight and Future Weight Gain: An fMRI Study," *Obesity (Silver Spring)* 19, no. 9 (September 2011): 1775–83; E. Stice et al., "Relation between Obesity and Blunted Striatal Response to Food Is Moderated by TaqIA A1 Allele," *Science* 322, no. 5900 (October 2008): 449–52; M. Naim et al., "Energy Intake, Weight Gain and Fat Deposition in Rats Fed Flavored, Nutritionally Controlled Diets in a Multichoice ('Cafeteria') Design," *Journal of Nutrition* 115, no. 11 (November 1985): 14447–58; R.J. Stubbs et al., "Effect of Altering the Variety of Sensorially Distinct Foods, of the Same Macronutrient Content, on Food Intake and Body Weight in Men," *European Journal of Clinical Nutrition* 55, no. 1 (January 2001): 19–28; J. Louis-Sylvestre et al., "Sensory versus Dietary Factors in Cafeteria-induced Overweight," *Physiology and Behavior* 32, no. 6 (June 1984): 901–5; J.D. Wene et al., "Flavor Preferences, Food Intake, and Weight Gain in Baboons," *Physiology and Behavior* 28, no. 3 (March 1982): 569–73.

11. J.H. Ledikwe, "A Reliable, Valid Questionnaire Indicates that

Preference for Dietary Fat Declines When Following a Reduced-fat Diet," *Appetite* 49, no. 1 (July 2007): 74–83.

12. Steven Heymsfield et al., "The Calorie: Myth, Measurement and Reality," *American Journal of Clinical Nutrition* 62, suppl. (1995): 1034S–41S; Klaas Westerterp, "The Assessment of Energy and Nutrient Intake in Humans," in Claude Bouchard, ed., *Physical Activity and Obesity* (Champaign, IL: Human Kinetics, 2000), 145; J.A. Tooze et al., "Psychosocial Predictors of Energy Underreporting in a Large Doubly Labeled Water Study," *American Journal of Clinical Nutrition* 79, no. 5 (2004): 795–804; D. Lansky and K. Brownell, "Estimates of Food Quantity and Calories: Errors in Self-report among Obese Patients," *American Journal of Clinical Nutrition* 35, no. 4 (1982): 727–32; M. Barbara et al., "Markers of the Validity of Reported Energy Intake," *Journal of Nutrition* 133, suppl. 3 (March 2003): 895S–920S.

13. David Kessler, *The End of Overeating: Taking Control of the Insatiable North American Appetite* (Toronto: McClelland and Stewart, 2009), 200.

7. GET MOTIVATED: GOAL SETTING AND THE SCIENCE OF BEHAVIOR CHANGE

1. E. Locke and G. Latham, "The Application of Goal Setting to Sports," *Journal of Sport Psychology* 7, no. 3 (September 1985): 205–22.

2. Roger Buehler et al., "Exploring the 'Planning Fallacy': Why People Underestimate Their Task Completion Times," *Journal of Personality and Social Psychology* 67, no. 3 (July 1994): 366–81.

3. C. Armitage and M. Conner, "Efficacy of the Theory of Planned Behavior: A Meta-analytic Review," *British Journal of Social Psychology* 40 (December 2001): 471–99.

4. Ibid.; Zan Gao and Maria Kosma, "Intention as a Mediator of Weight Training Behavior among College Students: An Integrative

Framework," *Journal of Applied Sport Psychology* 20 (2008):
363–74; J. Rise et al., "Predicting the Intention to Quit Smoking
and Quitting Behavior: Extending the Theory of Planned
Behaviour," *British Journal of Health Psychology* 13 (May 2008):
291–310; K. White et al., "Behavioral, Normative and Control
Beliefs Underlying Low-fat Dietary and Regular Physical Activity
Behaviors for Adults Diagnosed with Type 2 Diabetes and/or
Cardiovascular Disease," *Psychology, Health and Medicine* 12, no. 4
(August 2007): 485–94.

5.   Icek Ajzen, "From Intentions to Actions: A Theory of Planned
     Behavior," in Juliul Kuhl and Jürgen Beckman, eds., *Action Control:
     From Cognition to Behavior* (Berlin: Springer-Verlag, 1985), 12–13.

6.   Ibid., 22–25.

7.   Curt Lox et al., *The Psychology of Exercise: Integrating Theory and
     Practice* (Scottsdale, AZ: Holcomb Hathaway, 2006), 61.

8.   Albert Bandura, "Self-efficacy: Toward a Unifying Theory of
     Behavioral Change," *Psychological Review* 84 (March 1977): 191–215.

9.   B.F. Skinner, *Science and Human Behavior* (New York: Macmillan,
     1953), 65–66, 73.

10. Ibid., 70; Lox et al., *Psychology of Exercise,* 77–78.

11. Skinner, *Science and Human Behavior,* 70; Lox et al., *Psychology of
     Exercise,* 77–78.

12. Ibid., 78–79.

8. GET READY: MANAGING TIME, MONEY AND SOCIAL SUPPORT

1.   Paul Fuglestad et al., "Lifestyle Patterns Associated with Diet,
     Physical Activity, Body Mass Index and Amount of Recent Weight
     Loss in a Sample of Successful Weight Losers," *International Journal
     of Behavioral Nutrition and Physical Activity* 9:79 (June 2012): epub.

2.   "The Cross-platform Report, Q4, 2011," http://nielsen.com/us/
     en/insights/reports-downloads/2012/the-cross-platform-report-
     q4-2011.html. Accessed November 23, 2012.

3. "'Television Viewing," March 2006, http://www.statcan.gc.ca/daily-quotidien/060331/dq060331b-eng.htm. Accessed November 23, 2012.

4. Barbara Brehm, *Successful Fitness Motivation Strategies* (Champaign, IL: Human Kinetics, 2004), 65.

5. Mark Bittman, "Is Junk Food Really Cheaper?" *New York Times*, September 24, 2011.

6. Shauna Burke et al., "Group vs. Individual Approach: A Meta-analysis of the Effectiveness of Interventions to Promote Physical Activity," *Sport and Exercise Psychology Review* 2, no. 1 (February 2006): 19–35.

7. Megan Oaten and Ken Cheng, "Longitudinal Gains in Self-regulation from Regular Physical Exercise," *British Journal of Health Psychology* 11 (2006): 717–33.

8. Bronnie Ware, "Regrets of the Dying," http://www.inspirationand-chai.com/Regrets-of-the-Dying.html. Accessed November 17, 2012.

9. INTRODUCING THE VIRTUOUS CYCLE

1. Kathleen Vohs and Todd Heatherton, "Self-regulatory Failure: A Resource Depletion Approach," *Psychological Science* 11, no. 3 (May 2000): 249–54.

2. Roy Baumeister et al., "Ego Depletion: Is the Active Self a Limited Resource?" *Journal of Personality and Social Psychology* 74, no. 5 (May 1998): 1252–65.

3. M. Rosenkindle et al.,"Body Fat Loss and Compensatory Mechanisms in Response to Different Doses of Aerobic Exercise: A Randomized Controlled Trial in Overweight Sedentary Males," *American Journal of Physiology, Regulatory, Integrative and Comparative Physiology* 303, no. 6 (September 2012): R571–79.

4. David Kessler, *The End of Overeating: Taking Control of the Insatiable North American Appetite* (Toronto: McClelland and Stewart, 2009), 224.

5. Ibid., 221.
6. Yoni Freedhoff, "A Review of David Kessler's *The End of Overeating,*" March 22, 2010, http://www.weightymatters. ca/2010/03/review-of-david-kesslers-end-of.html. Accessed November 17, 2010.

10. THE VIRTUOUS CYCLE, LEVEL 1

1. "What Keeps You from Going to the Gym?" October 4, 2004, http://www.acefitness.org/pressroom/350/american-council-on-exercise-asks-1-500-web-site/. Accessed November 23, 2012.
2. "Artificial Sweeteners," MedicineNet, http://www.medicinenet. com/artificial_sweeteners/article.htm. Accessed November 22, 2012; B. Magnuson et al., "Aspartame: A Safety Evaluation Based on Current Use Levels, Regulations, and Toxicological and Epidemiological Studies," *Critical Reviews in Toxicology* 37, no. 8 (2007): 629–727; European Food Safety Authority, "Report of the Meetings on Aspartame with National Experts. Question Number: EFSA-Q-2009-00488," May 2010; H. Butchko et al., "Aspartame: Review of Safety," *Regulatory Toxicology and Pharmacology* 35, no. 2, pt. 2 (2002): S1–93; A. Otabe, "Advantame: An Overview of the Toxicity Data," *Food and Chemical Toxicology* 49, suppl. 1 (November 2011): S2–7.
3. US Food and Drug Administration, "Artificial Sweeteners: No Calories . . . Sweet!" *FDA Consumer Magazine*, July–August 2006.

11. THE VIRTUOUS CYCLE, LEVEL 2

1. Paul DeVita and Tibor Hortobágyi, "Obesity Is Not Associated with Increased Knee Joint Torque and Power during Level Walking," *Journal of Biomechanics* 9 (September 2003): 1355–62.
2. David Kessler, *The End of Overeating: Taking Control of the Insatiable*

North American Appetite (Toronto: McClelland and Stewart, 2009), 71–73.

12. THE VIRTUOUS CYCLE, LEVEL 3

1. An Pan et al., "Red Meat Consumption and Mortality: Results from 2 Prospective Cohort Studies," *Archives of Internal Medicine* 172, no. 7 (2012): 555–63; World Cancer Research Fund / American Institute for Cancer Research, "Food, Nutrition, Physical Activity, and the Prevention of Cancer: A Global Perspective," Washington, DC: AICR, 2007.
2. Teresa Fung et al., "Low-carbohydrate Diets and All-cause and Cause-specific Mortality: Two Cohort Studies," *Annals of Internal Medicine* 153, no. 5 (September 2010): 289–98.

APPENDIX A

1. "FDA Expands Warning to Consumers about Tainted Weight Loss Pills; List Increases from 28 to 69 Products; Agency Seeking Recalls," http://www.fda.gov/newsevents/newsroom/pressannouncements/2008/ucm116998.htm. Accessed November 17, 2012.

APPENDIX B

1. "Large Scale Analysis Finds Bariatric Surgery Relatively Safe," http://www.dukehealth.org/health_library/news/large_scale_analysis_finds_bariatric_surgery_relatively_safe. Accessed November 9, 2012.

APPENDIX C

1. Beth Abramovitz and Leann Birch, "Five-year-old Girls' Ideas about Dieting Are Predicted by Their Mothers' Dieting," *Journal of the American Dietetic Association* 100, no. 10 (October 2000): 1157–63.
2. Ibid.

RESOURCES

www.BodyForWife.com – This is my personal website where you can get a free Metabolism Report as well as a free book of recipes that are lower in calories and easy to make.

Nancy Clark, *Nancy Clark's Sport Nutrition Guidebook*, Human Kinetics, 4th Edition, 2008. – This is a great book for helping you adopt the "food as fuel" for exercise performance mind-set.

www.Fitocracy.com – I have not personally used this site, but I have heard good things about it as a fitness social network to help motivate people to exercise. A warning that there may be fitness advice shared on this site that is not safe or advisable.

Dr. David Kessler, *The End of Overeating*, Rodale, 2009. – Although I suggested in chapter 9 that Dr. Kessler's "all or none" approach to food rehab is wrong, this is still a great book for its exposé of the food industry.

www.SixPackAbs.com – It may seem strange to promote such a website in this book, but I am co-founder of this site and you can find a lot of my writing here. I cover a wide variety of fitness subjects for all shapes, sizes and genders. However, I'll warn you that it's not always politically correct.

Lisa Young, *The Portion Teller*, Crown Archetype, 2005. – For people who must eat at restaurants frequently due to travel and business lunches, this book can be a valuable tool for lowering your caloric intake while dining out.

LIST OF INTERVIEWS

Anna Mae Alexander

Miguel Alonso-Alonso, MD, instructor in neurology, Harvard Medical School

James Annesi, PhD, director of wellness and advancement, YMCA Metro Atlanta

Alan Aragon, MSc (nutrition), independent nutrition expert, Los Angeles

Sean Astin, actor

Nicole Avena, PhD, research neuroscientist, University of Florida / Princeton University

Daniel Baldwin, actor

Jessica Banas, office worker

Barney Barnowski, business development manager

Marty Becker, DVM, veterinarian for VetStreet.com and author

Cathy Beddia, pharmaceutical company employee

Kris Beneteau, office worker

Hans-Rudolf Berthoud, PhD, George H. Bray professor, Neurobiology of Nutrition Laboratory, Pennington Biomedical Research Center, Baton Rouge, Louisiana

Cheryl Berube, graphic designer

Michael Biehn, actor

Darlene Bordin, accountant

Emma Boyland, PhD, research associate in biopsychology, University of Liverpool

Bruce Bradley, MBA, former food company marketing executive and author

Bert Carron, PhD, professor of kinesiology, University of Western Ontario, London, Ontario

Stacy Lynn Carter, administrative assistant

Charlene Casey, records manager

Tim Church, MD, PhD, professor, John S. McIlHenny Endowed Chair
in Health Wisdom, Pennington Biomedical Research Center

Liz Claman, national news anchor

Nancy Clark, MSc, RD, sport nutrition expert and author

Chandra Crawford, Olympic champion cross-country skier

Wes Daniel, property manager

Carolyn Davis, PhD, professor, Faculty of Health, York University

Irene Davis, PhD, professor, director, Spaulding National Running
Center, Harvard Medical School

Jennifer Dewey, fitness director at the Betty Ford Center in Rancho
Mirage, California

Charlene Elliot, PhD, associate professor of food marketing, University
of Calgary

Avery Faigenbaum, PhD, professor of health and exercise science, the
College of New Jersey

Heidi Fell, MD, family physician and amazing, brilliant, beautiful wife

Reed Ferber, PhD, assistant professor of biomechanics, director,
Running Injury Clinic, University of Calgary

Maryanne Fisher, PhD, professor of psychology, St. Mary's University

Yoni Freedhoff, MD, assistant professor of family medicine, University
of Ottawa, founder, Bariatric Medical Institute

Chris Frolek, RN

Harish Ganesh, entrepreneur

Leeza Gibbons

Leigh Gibson, PhD, professor of biopsychology, University of
Roehampton, London, UK

Eric Goebelbecker, dog trainer and computer programmer

Peter Gollwitzer, PhD, professor of psychology, New York University

Matt Grevers, Olympic champion swimmer

Jen Hamel, personal trainer

Mark Heard, MD, orthopedic surgeon, Banff Mineral Springs Hospital

Mariel Hemingway, actor

Clara Hughes, Olympic champion, speed skating and cycling

Michael Joyner, MD, physician-researcher, Mayo Clinic, Rochester, Minnesota

David Katz, MD, director, Yale University Prevention Research Center

Adam Van Koeverden, Olympic champion flat-water kayaker

Bill Kohl, PhD, professor of epidemiology and kinesiology, University of Texas

Vasilios Kosteas, PhD, associate professor of economics, Cleveland State University

Elaine LaLanne, fitness entrepreneur

Jenna Lee, journalist and national news anchor

Lynn Leroux

Graham Levy, electronic technician

Richard Mattes, PhD, RD, distinguished professor of nutrition science, Purdue University

Teri McCambridge, MD, director of sports medicine, Cincinnati Children's Hospital, associate professor of pediatrics, University of Cincinnati

Jen McKinnon

Sarah McLachlan, singer and songwriter

Kris McParland, corporate manager

Katrina Mealey, PhD, associate professor of veterinary medicine, Washington State University

Cesar Millan, dog trainer and television personality

Gordon Patzer, PhD, author and professor of business administration, Roosevelt University, Illinois

Neil Peart, drummer, Rush

Sue Pedersen, MD, specialist in endocrinology and metabolism, Calgary

Stuart Phillips, PhD, professor of kinesiology, McMaster University, Hamilton, Ontario

Stefan Pinto, model and entrepreneur

Eric Ravussin, PhD, professor and Chief, Division of Health and Performance Enhancement, Pennington Biomedical Research Center

Raylene Reimer, PhD, RD, associate professor of nutrition, University
of Calgary

Susan Sadler

Peter Sargious, MD, medical director, chronic disease management,
Alberta Health Services

Jane Schmidt, grocery store employee

Marty Scott, city planner

Tony Sekullich, television writer

Jane Seymour, actor

Chris Shandley, global account executive

Nia Shanks, personal trainer, co-founder, Girls Gone Strong

Arya Sharma, MD, professor of medicine and chair in obesity research
and management at the University of Alberta, founder and scientific director of the Canadian Obesity Network

Michael Shermer, PhD, founding publisher of *Skeptic* magazine, executive director of the Skeptic's Society, adjunct professor, Claremont
Graduate University and Chapman University, Orange, California

Kyle Shewfelt, Olympic champion gymnast

Jen Sinkler, editorial director of fitness content for *Experience Life*
magazine

Brent Smith, singer, Shinedown

Paul Stanley, singer and guitar player, KISS

Eric Stice, PhD, research scientist, Oregon Research Institute

Jim Taylor, PhD, author and adjunct professor in sport psychology,
University of San Francisco

Michelle Voss, PhD, assistant professor of psychology, University of Iowa

Margriet Westerterp, PhD, professor of regulation of food intake,
University of Maastricht

Montel Williams, talk show host

Wendy Williams, talk show host

Lisa Young, PhD, RD, author and adjunct professor of nutrition, New
York University

Margaret Yutera-Leitch, PhD, author, obesity research and adjunct
professor, University of Calgary

INDEX

JAMES FELL is the author of the syndicated column "In-Your-Face Fitness" for the *Chicago Tribune,* and interviews celebrities about their fitness regimens for the *Los Angeles Times.* He is senior fitness columnist for Chatelaine.com and AskMen.com. He has published more than 100 articles with AOL as the "Fit Family Guy." Fell lives in Calgary, Alberta, where he also works as a fitness consultant.

www.BodyForWife.com and www.SixPackAbs.com

MARGARET YÚFERA-LEITCH is an obesity researcher and adjunct professor in the University of Calgary's Faculty of Kinesiology. She has published peer-reviewed journal articles in the field of eating behavior, and is a contributing author for *Impulse* and *Fat Planet.* She lives in Calgary, Alberta.

www.PsychologyOfAppetite.com